Cooking for Health

Arthritis

Macrobiotic Food and Cooking Series

MACROBIOTIC FOOD AND COOKING SERIES

Cooking for Health

Arthritis

by Aveline Kushi

edited by Wendy Esko

foreword by David Dodson, M.D.

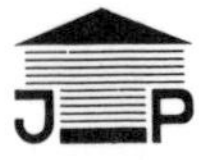

Japan Publications, Inc.
Tokyo · New York

Note to the reader: Those with health problems are advised to seek the guidance of a qualified medical, or psychological professional in addition to that of a qualified macrobiotic counselor before implementing any of the dietary and other approaches presented in this book. It is essential that any reader who has any reason to suspect serious illness in themselves or their family members seek appropriate medical, nutritional, or psychological advice promptly. Neither this or any other health related book should be used as a substitute for qualified care or treatment.

Published by Japan Publications, Inc., Tokyo and New York

Distributors:
United States: *Kodansha International/USA, Ltd., through Harper & Row, Publishers, Inc., 599 Lexington Avenue, Suite 2300, New York, N. Y. 10022.* South America: *Harper & Row, Publishers, Inc., International Department.* Canada: *Fitzhenry & Whiteside Ltd., 195 Allstate Parkway, Markham, Ontario, L3R 4T8.* Mexico and Central America: *HARLA S. A. de C. V., Apartado 30–546, Mexico 4, D. F.* British Isles: *Premier Book Marketing Ltd., 1 Gower Street, London WC1E 6HA.* European Continent: *European Book Service PBD, Strijkviertel 63, 3454 PK De Meern, The Netherlands.* Australia and New Zealand: *Bookwise International, 54 Crittenden Road, Findon, South Australia 5007.* The Far East and Japan: *Japan Publications Trading Co., Ltd., 1–2–1, Sarugaku-cho, Chiyoda-ku, Tokyo 101.*

First edition: November 1988

LCCC No. 86–081323
ISBN 0–87040–677–9

Printed in U.S.A.

Foreword

Just over one-hundred years ago, the notion that invisible, microscopic "germs" caused disease would have been considered completely crackpot. By the 1880s though, brilliant men such as Lister, Pasteur, and Koch had conclusively demonstrated that microbes do indeed cause numerous conditions including tuberculosis, malaria, and even leprosy. Today many people doubt the link between diet and health, particularly doctors! In fact, the Arthritis Foundation recently distributed a pamphlet which stated, "The truth about diet and arthritis may surprise you. It is simply this: There is no special diet for arthritis. No specific food has anything to do with causing it. And no specific diet will cure it."

Even the Arthritis Foundation no longer believes this nonsense, but nevertheless, many doctors still believe that diet plays only a minor role, if any at all, in arthritis, or in most other conditions for that matter. Let us briefly examine why I referred to the above quote as nonsense.

First of all, arthritis means inflammation of joints. Medicine now recognizes about one-hundred different types of arthritis—rheumatoid arthritis, gout, and post-traumatic arthritis are just three examples. No matter what type of arthritis you have though, the more you weigh, the more your joints are likely to hurt. If you have a sore knee or ankle, you surely will not want to carry a fifty-pound sack of flour around. Unfortunately, overweight arthritics carry around pounds they cannot get rid of as easily as setting down a sack of flour. Macrobiotics is definitely the ultimate weight-loss diet, and solving any weight problem will automatically make the overweight arthritic more comfortable.

There are at least two other mechanisms by which a macrobiotic diet can help arthritis sufferers. The first deals with a group of substances known as *autocoids*, or locally acting hormones. The best known autocoids are the *prostaglandins*. There are numerous different types of prostaglandins produced throughout the body which regulate inflammation and other vital functions. The prostaglandins ultimately derive from the food we eat and therefore, by changing the kinds of food we eat, we also change the prostaglandins and other autocoids in our bodies. This has been shown to have a beneficial effect on arthritis as reported in Britain's prestigious medical journal *The Lancet*, on January 26, 1985. More specifically, it appears that animal fats are converted into the types of prostaglandins that increase inflammation.

Finally, there is the issue of food allergy. Food allergy is an extremely confusing issue in medicine, so confusing in fact, that many doctors do not believe it exists. This is principally because the symptoms of food allergy can occur up to three weeks after eating the offending food and because many, if not most, patients are allergic to not just one but to several foods. Thus, if Mary has arthritis caused by allergy to eggs, milk, and tomatoes, and she eliminates eggs and milk but not tomatoes, she may fail to get better and may mistakenly believe she is not allergic to milk and eggs. Furthermore, if Mary were careful not to consume any eggs, milk, or tomatoes for two weeks and failed to get better, she might conclude erroneously—though not unreasonably—that she was not allergic to these foods. As mentioned above, allergic symptoms may not occur for up to three weeks after eating the allergen, or allergy-causing substance.

It has now been clearly demonstrated that several types of arthritis are related to food allergy. Interestingly, the first reliable report in the medical literature was a report which appeared in the *Annals of Allergy* in 1969. The author of the article, Dr. Stephan Epstein, had carefully documented the fact that his own case of palindromic rheumatism was caused by allergy to peppermint and to nitrites, a common food additive. It is curious that this fascinating and thorough report failed to convince more doctors of the importance of food allergy, particularly considering that the author and patient was himself a physician!

The macrobiotic diet avoids the common food allergens: milk, eggs, and sugar are the "big three." As illustrated by Dr. Epstein's case, food additives can be the allergen in some cases, and therefore the macrobiotic principle of using only the best quality, organic foods is also important for those who suffer from arthritis and other conditions that may be caused by food allergy. A warning though: you may find you are allergic to some good macrobiotic foods. For example, fish and strawberries, either of which can be consumed occasionally by most macrobiotic people, are two fairly common food allergens.

I hope this brief discussion serves to dispell the old idea most doctors were taught in medical school that diet has nothing to do with arthritis. Diet has much to do with arthritis and perhaps most other diseases as well. As a physician and a nutritionist, I see the connection in terms of allergies, autocoids, and so on. To the macrobiotic teacher, the connection may be expressed in terms of the traditional Oriental view. To look at the subject both ways is to see the Yin and the Yang, to see the big picture. It is only by looking at the big picture that we can hope to successfully deal with big problems, such as the problem of arthritis.

David Dodson, M.D.
Boston, Massachusetts

Preface

The problem of arthritis is widespread today. It is usually associated with aging, and some people may even consider it a normal part of growing older.

However, the idea that our body should become stiff, painful, and inflexible as we get older is incorrect. The experiences of long-lived peoples such as the Hunza in Pakistan and the Tarahumara in Mexico prove that a flexible, active, and productive old age is possible when we live in harmony with the laws of nature. These people remain active into their nineties (some live to be well over one hundred) with no arthritis, rheumatism, or other conditions normally associated with aging. Their diet is essentially macrobiotic: it is based around whole cereal grains, beans, fresh local vegetables, and other regional foods.

Macrobiotic friends are also normally very supple and flexible. However, some friends have noticed that the flexibility of their joints and muscles changes from day to day depending on what they eat. Friends who have eaten too much fish or other animal food sometimes report feeling more stiff and inflexible on the following day. Overeating or a lack of chewing can also produce a similar effect.

More and more, scientific research is linking the way we eat with a variety of disorders, including arthritis and related joint problems. A traditional, ecologically based diet can help in the prevention of these problems, and can help people with arthritis regain bodily flexibility. It is my hope that the recipes and menus presented in this simple introductory book can help guide everyone in the direction of a more balanced diet for increased health, vitality, and flexibility.

I would like to thank our friends who assisted in completing this book. I thank our long-time friend and associate, Wendy Esko, for compiling and editing the text. I also thank Edward Esko for reviewing the manuscript, and for suggesting the application of the five transformations of energy to the problem of arthritis.

I also thank Charles Millman for completing Michio Kushi's companion volume in the *Macrobiotic Health Education Series*, and thank Dr. David Dodson for writing a foreword.

I would also like to thank Lillian Kushi, Christian Gautier, Jay Kelly, and other friends for their efforts in illustrating the *Food and Cooking Series*, and thank Susi Ostrreich for typing the text.

I also thank Mr. Iwao Yoshizaki and Mr. Yoshiro Fujiwara, respectively president and New York representative of Japan Publications, Inc., for their dedication to making many fine books on macrobiotics available, including the books in this series.

Finally, I thank our friend Phillip Jannetta, currently living in Tokyo, for doing the editorial work on this book.

Aveline Kushi
Brookline, Massachusetts
July, 1987

Contents

1. The Source of Health

The quality of our life—whether we are sick or healthy, happy or unhappy, at peace or disturbed—depends on the quality of the factors that we take in from the environment, near and far.

We, all human beings, exist at the center of a huge spiral that encompasses all of the dimensions of our environment, both natural and man-made. These factors are constantly changing, and ultimately, transforming themselves into human life through a process of universal materialization. When we see this process from the perspective of the universe, we can say that these factors are becoming more and more condensed, as they spiral in toward human life. When we see this process from our human perspective, we can say that we attract or take in the multitude of factors from our environment.

The dimensions of our environmental spiral encompass both visible and invisible worlds. Among the visible aspects are air, water, soil, light, and the many nutritional factors taken in daily in the form of food. Invisible factors include various forms of radiation, energy, and waves that emanate from the far reaches of the universe.

Today, everyone is concerned with the quality of life. We know that a clean, natural environment, including fresh air, natural sunlight, fresh vegetation, and clean water is essential to health and well-being. We are able to control or be selective in the quality of these factors by choosing a certain living place, occupation, leisure activity, and in other ways.

The more obscure, invisible components of our environment,

Fig. 1 The Spiral of Health

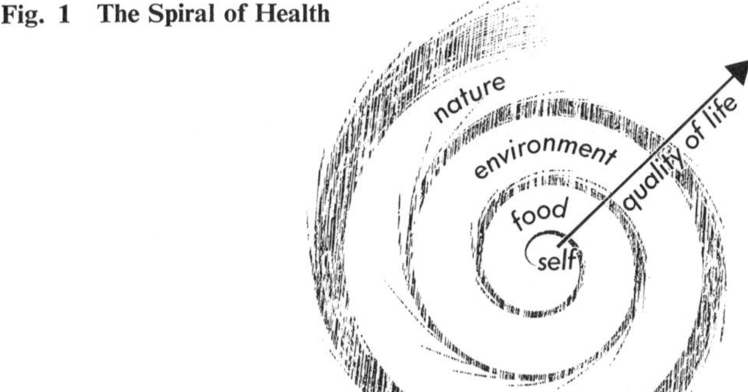

including various forms of energy and natural radiation, are continually streaming in toward the planet, and are more or less beyond our control. However, through our choice of food and through activities such as meditation, we are able to emphasize certain vibrational qualities while de-emphasizing others.

The environmental factor over which we have the most control is our daily food. We can see our daily food and drink as the condensed essence of our larger environment, the form from which our biological makeup is constructed.

Our physical and emotional health, and the overall quality of our life, is determined largely by the quality of our daily food. Moment to moment, new cells, body fluids, and tissues are formed out of what we eat and drink. We are, in a sense, phantoms of our daily foods.

Macrobiotics recognizes the all-important role of daily food, along with factors such as activity, attitude, and lifestyle in determining the quality of our life and health. It emphasizes the selection of the highest quality foods and beverages for the purpose of creating the most natural quality of life, including sound physical and mental health.

In the introductory sections that follow, we explain the underlying principles of macrobiotics, including the universal spiral of life and the balancing principle of yin and yang.

Throughout the world, hundreds of thousands of people have adopted a macrobiotic way of life and have experienced improved health. The dietary principles of macrobiotics can be used to prevent the various forms of arthritis, as well as other degenerative diseases that affect millions of people in the world today. At the same time, they can be adopted by people with bone and joint conditions as a method for health improvement. It is our hope that in the future, the approach to arthritis and related conditions will involve an assessment of each person's dietary practice along with recommendations for the improvement of diet and way of life.

The Underlying Principles

There is a vast cosmology behind the principles of macrobiotics, a cosmology which sets out to explain the creation and the interrelationship of all phenomena throughout the universe.

The real purpose of macrobiotics is to empower us with the ability to fulfill our potentials and dreams, and to serve as a reminder that we are the builders and masters of our own lives.

Macrobiotics is a rich and unlimited field of study that extends far beyond the scope of this book. Readers are encouraged to investigate the infinite application of the macrobiotic principles, which are also called the Unifying Principles. In doing so, individuals can become their own guide, discovering for themselves what is needed to maintain health and to accomplish personal goals. This chapter contains a brief overview of the macrobiotic principles and how they apply to the particular subjects of diet and health. For more detailed information, and for examples of applying the Unifying Principles to other areas, readers are referred to any of the variety of books listed in the bibliography.

Everything in the universe is a constantly moving and changing energy, varying in density and speed. Even seemingly stable and solid objects, a rock or a table for instance, are made up of moving molecules, atoms, electrons and protons, which themselves are nothing but energy.

When moving in a yang (△) direction, energy begins to take on form in a process of materialization. Generally speaking, this process is characterized by increasing speed, increasing temperature, and more density and weight, which manifest as compactness or contraction. When moving in a yin (▽) direction, energy takes on the opposite characteristics. It is slower, cooler, more diffused, expanded, and lighter in weight. Yang motion is followed by yin, and yin motion is followed by yang. Yang does not exist without yin, nor yin without yang.

Human beings, as the end result of a yang, centripetal spiral, are also at the beginning of a yin, centrifugal spiral. As we develop in a more yang direction, we are created by physical food, the elemental energies from the sun, water, wind, and so on, and the vibrations of thoughts from the mind. After we are formed in the physical world, we start to grow in the opposite, or yin direction, as we develop emotionally, mentally, and spiritually. Eventually, our physical body

The deeper meaning of health is being in this aligned and harmonious state which results in a smooth, unblocked, effortless flow of our energies between all the inner and outer universal parts of ourselves. The macrobiotic approach to well-being is a holistic approach directed by our understanding that a change in any aspect or portion of our body or self has an effect on everything else including the world and the universe. There are several approaches one can take to create a free flow of energy:

1. *Dietary changes:* This is the perspective that this book basically focuses on. What we eat creates our blood cells, and hence the formation of our organs and all other parts of our body. It is a wonder that food is not often associated as a major cause of

disease. One's diet also alters the mind and emotions. We know that the ingestion of alcohol and various licit and illicit drugs effects one's mental state. This fact cannot be argued. Likewise, anything else one takes in has its effect on our being, though it may be on a subtle level.

2. *Working with the powers of the mind:* Everything that exists has its origin in the invisible world of the mind and vibrations. It is said that what we believe manifests. There are many negative thoughts or assumptions that we may dwell on which can influence our lives. Many of these delusions, as we may call them here, occur automatically and unconsciously. One may develop self-awareness by constantly observing the thoughts, actions, and reactions that control one's life and rechannel unwanted habits into more positive ideas and dreams.

3. *Relaxation:* Mental and physical tension block the freest flow of energy. A technique one may try is to take an inventory of all the parts of your body and relax all tense spots. You can do the same thing with the mind, letting go of anxiety, guilt and anger. Use the breath to help the relaxation process: breathe slowly and deeply.

4. *Palm-healing and shiatsu massage:* These practices can be used to temporarily unblock stagnations of energy in the body.

5. *Keep mentally and physically active:* Exercise, do sports or dancing, clean your house, garden, read, study, engage in hobbies, draw, write, compose, play music, do volunteer work, teach . . . whatever you want. Make sure to do both mental and physical work. The more energy we circulate, the more comes back to us and the less stagnation there is in our lives.

6. *Changing one's environmental surroundings:* In some cases, it might be necessary to change one's environmental surroundings. Some forms of sickness can be more easily eliminated in a warm climate while others may require cooler temperatures. Moving to a quieter locale may be beneficial for some conditions. Also, it is important that one be in a loving atmosphere with people who care about us and support us. We can help maintain a clean, ecologically balanced environment by using biodegradable products and materials, by not taking more than we need, and by

helping to protect the well-being of our fellow inhabitants on this earth—the members of the plant and animal kingdoms.

7. *Maintaining good relations with all the people in our lives:* Blaming, holding grudges, the emotions of anger, fear, and hatred, make one very tense and cause blockages. We create the circumstances of our individual lives so it is up to us to change them. Give everyone the emotions of love, support, and respect for their freedom and individuality.

8. *Being grateful for all that we have been given:* Notice all the beauty and marvels in the world. Look at hardships, difficulties, or rejections as opportunities for self-reflection and growth.

Working on just one of the above recommendations can be tremendously helpful and have a positive effect on us overall. However, to make a really permanent and thorough change for the better, all of the above should be worked on, as they are interrelated. Many people

Yin and Yang

Everything is created and governed by the interactions of yin and yang, the two opposite poles which are endlessly manifesting in the world. The chart below lists some classification examples.

By learning how yin and yang relate to each other you can begin to understand all the workings of the world. The chart on the next page lists some classification examples. Two basic tendencies of yin and yang are:

Yin attracts yang and yang attracts yin, resulting in the harmony and marriage of two opposites. Examples are: man and woman, plus and minus magnets or electrical charges, electron and proton, spirit and matter, and so on. Upon injesting a quantity of salt (yang) for instance, one is then attracted to liquids (yin).

Yin repels yin, yang repels yang. Examples are: oil and water (both yin) do not mix. Two plus poles repel each other as do two minus poles.

Let us look at a few more examples of yin and yang from everyday life. When we become hungry, our stomach becomes more yang or contracted. We naturally seek food in order to make our digestive vessels more expanded, or yin. After eating, we are no longer attracted to food,.an example of yin repelling yin. When we are very

Attribute	Yin/Centrifugal (▽)	Yang/Centripetal(△)
Tendency	Expansion	Contraction
Function	Dispersion, decomposition	Assimilation, organization
Movement	More inactive, slower	More active, faster
Vibration	Shorter waves, high frequency	Longer waves, low frequency
Direction	Vertical, ascending	Horizontal, descending
Position	More outward and peripheral	More inward and central
Weight	Lighter	Heavier
Temperature	Colder	Hotter
Light	Darker	Lighter
Humidity	More wet	More dry
Density	Thinner	Thicker
Size	Larger	Smaller
Shape	More expanded, fragile	More contracted, harder
Length	Longer	Shorter
Texture	Softer	Harder
Atomic particle	Electron	Proton
Elements	N, O, K, P, Ca	H, C, Na, As, Mg
Environment	Vibration→Air→Water→	Earth
Climate	Tropical	Arctic
Biology	Vegetable	Animal
Sex	Female	Male
Organ structure	Hollow, expansive	Compact, condensed
Nerves	Orthosympathetic	Parasympathetic
Attitude	Gentle, negative	Active, positive
Work	Psychological & mental	Physical & social
Consciousness	More universal	More specific
Mental function	Dealing with the future	Dealing with the past
Culture	Spiritually oriented	Materially oriented
Color	Purple→Blue→Green→ Yellow→	Brown→Orange→Red
Season	Winter	Summer
Dimension	Space	Time
Taste	Hot→sour→sweet→	Salty→Bitter
Vitamins	C	K, D
Catalyst	Water	Fire

active, or more yang, we naturally seek rest, a more yin condition, and after resting, we again seek activity.

When we travel somewhere, we do so because we are attracted to something in the environment that is new and different from the place in which we live, a case of opposites attracting. Once we experience many things in the new environment, we are naturally attracted to the more familiar environment of home.

When we write something with a pen, the more dry and rough surface of the paper, which is more yang, attracts the moist ink which is more yin. However, if the paper becomes more yin, for example, wet or coated with wax, it is much more difficult to write on.

The burning of wood in a fireplace offers yet another example of yin and yang. The more yang fire is attracted to the more yin wood, and so it burns. The ash, which represents the more yang residue left after the more yin parts of the wood turn into gases, gradually falls off or crumbles, an example of yang repelling yang.

When we enroll in a school, be it the Kushi Institute or Harvard University, we do so because we are attracted to what it has to offer, which we perceive as something that we lack. Then, after studying for a certain period, we absorb what the school has to offer, and at some point, are no longer attracted to it but are instead attracted to the world outside. This example illustrates the principle of opposites attracting initially, and then, as they become more like each other, repelling one another.

As we can see, yin and yang are dynamic, always changing into each other as the ceaseless movement of life continues.

The force of attraction (or repulsion as the case may be) is proportional to the ratio of the yin and yang elements. Their combination in various proportions creates an infinite variety of energies and phenomena where no two things in existence are identical.

Yin and yang are not static and are always flowing from one to another in various degrees. Yin in the extreme changes to yang and vice versa. Nothing lasts forever. Day turns into night, night into day. Activity is followed by rest, rest by activity. Success follows failure and failure follows success. Civilizations rise and fall. What has a beginning has an end.

Nothing is totally yin or totally yang. All things are made up of both. The more yin something is, the more yang it is as well. Many people that appear yang, strong, rough and tough on the outside may in comparison be yin, weak, and fragile on the inside. Others that appear yin, soft, and fragile on the outside may well be yang, strong and stubborn on the inside. Something that is structurally yang, as is the dense and compacted liver, is energetically yin; it functions without much motion. Things that are structurally yin, as is the hollow heart, are energetically more yang, as it never stops pumping, contracting and expanding. The bigger the front, the bigger the back.

Large yin attracts small yin, large yang attracts small yang. After you take sugar (large yin) you are drawn to drinking more fluids (small yin).

Yin creates yang, yang creates yin. A yin, colder climate creates yang, small, hardy vegetation and a more yang, ambitious, hard-driving society. While a yang, warmer climate creates yin, watery, large, lush vegetation and a more slow paced, easy going and relaxed society.

Everything on this earth is created by varying proportions of upward and downward energies. Gravity is an example of downward energy. The growth of trees and plants is an example of upward energy.

Yin and Yang and Diet

Yang foods give warmth, strength, discipline, and vitality. Excessively yang foods (such as red meat, eggs, or too much salt) are known to cause tightness and hardness in the body and mind, including rigidity, egocentricity, exclusivity, restlessness, violent tendencies, and certain types of cancer, arthritic conditions, and so on.

Yin foods are cooling, cleansing, relaxing, and nurture patience and understanding. Excessively yin foods (such as honey, sugar, chemicals, and drugs) have been shown to cause weakening and dispersion of the functioning capabilities in body and mind, including fear, defensiveness, loss of will, susceptibility to viruses, a rampage of white-blood-cell production, and depression or suicidal tendencies, to name some common problems.

When taking in overly yang foods, one is automatically attracted to overly yin ones (and vice versa) to make balance and compensation. One may end up on a wild or chaotic seesaw with a combination of unwanted side effects such as the ones listed above. Macrobiotics recommends a diet of more centrally balanced foods. Grains are the most centered and appropriate foods for human beings, requiring only a minimum amount of counterbalancing. (Grains are our complementary opposites as they are the last stage of plant evolution just as we are the last stage of animal evolution.) Brown rice, especially, has the right proportion of yin and yang factors for humans, and provides the most stabilizing dietary staple.

Humans are constitutionally yang, warm-blooded beings, and therefore require most if not all of their nourishment from their complementary opposite, which is the yin, vegetable kingdom. Among animal foods, fish is the recommended choice, particularly slow moving, white-meat varieties, as well as some types of shellfish. The human digestive system does not digest or assimilate meat well. It lingers and putrefies in the lower digestive tract. The only circumstance where it is healthy to eat large amounts of animal food is in

Fig. 2 General Yin (▽) and Yang (△) Categories of Foods

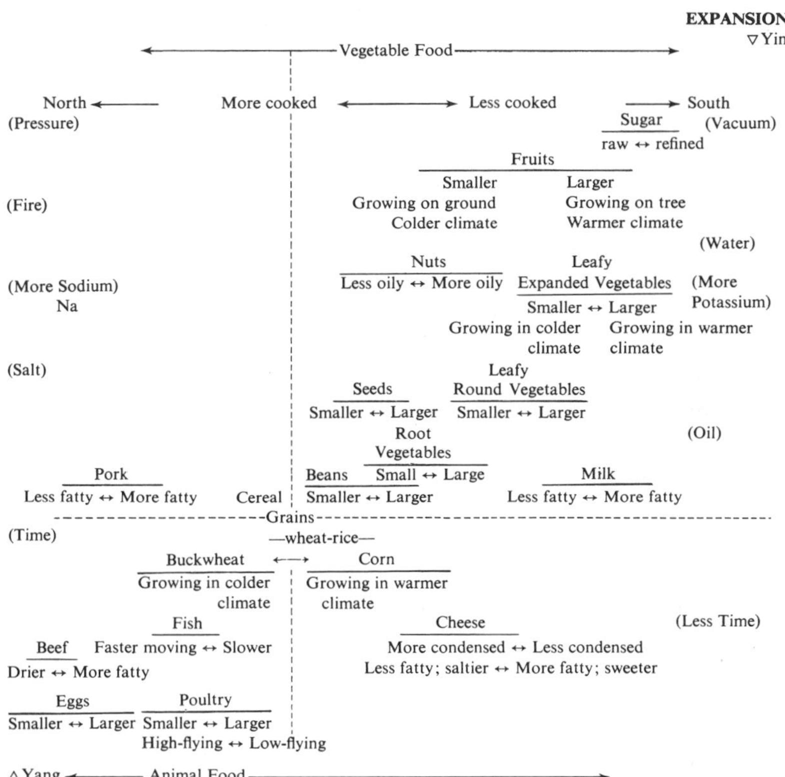

The above chart gives the general classification of food groups from yang to yin. However, more precise classification should be made upon examination of environmental conditions, nature and structure, chemical compounds, and effect upon our physical and mental conditions. Also, cooking can greatly change food qualities from yin to yang and yang to yin.

the very cold, yin, arctic regions where more strongly yang food is needed and where the availability of plant food is minimal.

Actually, climate plays a major role in our choice of food. It is recommended that we choose fresh produce which is grown or can grow in our own climatic zone. Tropical fruits are more appropriate when consumed where they are grown. They are detrimental to one's health when taken in large quantities, or too often, in the temperate zone.

The progression of the seasons also plays an important part in food selection. For instance, in the spring, when the energy is rising and expanding, we should include fresh young greens and sprouts in our meals. Towards fall and then winter, when the energies are descending and contracting, squash, kale, and winter-storable vegetables such as root vegetables, and dried plants such as sea vegetables should be consumed.

A variety of cooking methods should be employed as well. In the winter, we can eat more well-cooked, slightly saltier, pressure-cooked, and baked foods, as well as more fish. In the summer, more lightly cooked, boiled, raw (such as salads and fruits), chilled, and steamed foods and desserts may be consumed.

Also, within one meal we should ideally have a representative variety of cooking styles, as well as a variety of tastes, colors, and sizes.

Two additional factors which determine what is yin and what is yang, and to what relative degree, are: (1) rate of growth (faster is more yin and slower is more yang), and (2) the portion of the plant being considered—whether roots (more yang) or leaves and fruits (more yin).

Figure 4 represents a general yin/yang categorization of foods. (Reprinted from the *Book of Macrobiotics: The Universal Way of Health and Happiness* by Michio Kushi, p. 57.)

2. Explanation of the Standard Macrobiotic Diet

The dietary recommendations that make up the Standard Macrobiotic Diet are suggested for individuals in a generally sound state of health.

Fig. 3 Standard Macrobiotic Diet*

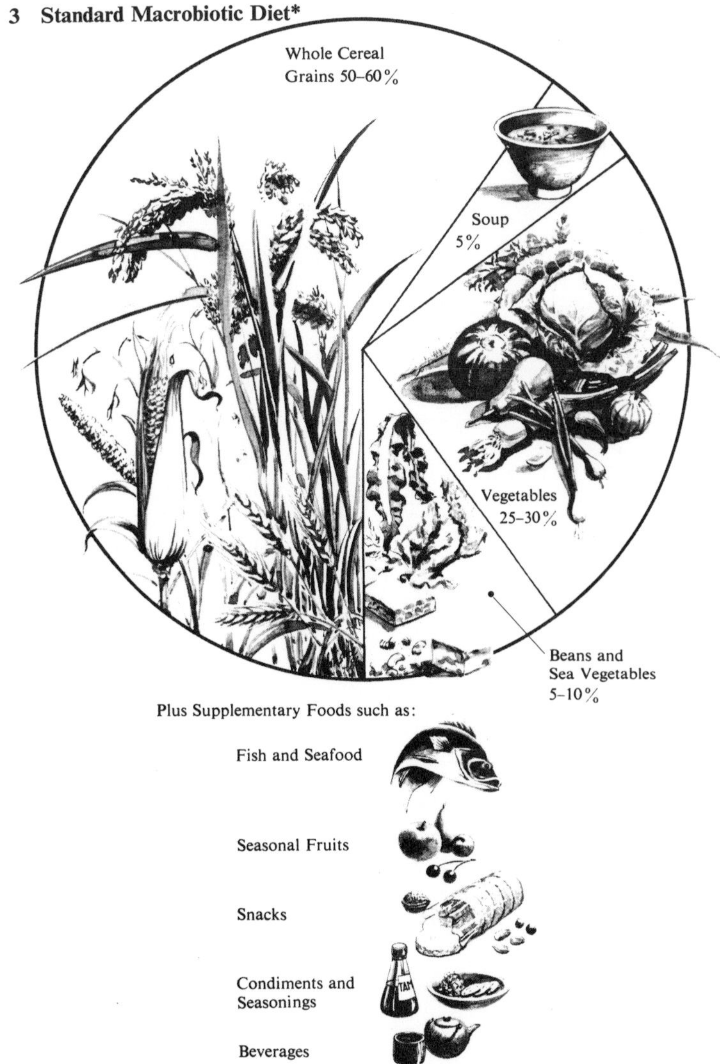

Persons having a more serious condition may need further modifications. It should also be noted that this is a general guideline and that whatever one's state of health, each person's individuality, life-style, and environment need to be taken into account with the diet adapted accordingly.

To see exactly what foods are recommended, refer to the detailed food list following the section below on proportions.

1. WHOLE CEREAL GRAINS. It is recommended that at least 50 percent of every meal include cooked, organically grown, whole cereal grains prepared in a variety of ways.

2. SOUPS. Approximately 5 to 10 percent of daily food intake (one or two bowls daily) may include soup made with traditional and naturally processed *miso* or *tamari* soy sauce. The flavor should not be overly salty, and soups may include a variety of grains, beans, and vegetables, including sea vegetables such as *wakame* and *kombu*.

3. VEGETABLES. About 20 to 30 percent of each meal may include local and organically grown vegetables with a large amount cooked in various styles and a smaller amount eaten as raw salad.

4. BEANS AND SEA VEGETABLES. Approximately 5 to 10 percent of the daily diet may include cooked beans and sea vegetables.

   Sea vegetables may be prepared in a variety of ways. They can be cooked with beans or vegetables, used in soups, or cooked and eaten separately as side dishes, flavored with a moderate amount of tamari soy sauce, sea salt, or rice vinegar.

5. SUPPLEMENTARY FOODS. Foods in the supplementary category may comprise approximately 5 to 10 percent of a meal. Once or twice weekly, a small amount of fresh white-meat fish may be eaten if desired.

   Fruit desserts, including fresh and dried fruits, may also be consumed on occasion. Local and organically grown fruits are preferred. Frequent use of fruit juice is not advisable. However, occasional consumption in warmer weather is allowable, depending on our health.

   Lightly roasted seeds may be enjoyed as a snack. Though less frequently, some roasted nuts may be consumed. Rice syrup and barley malt may be used occasionally to add a sweet taste; rice vinegar or *umeboshi* vinegar may also be used occasionally for a sour taste.

6. BEVERAGES. Any traditional tea which does not have an aromatic fragrance or a stimulant effect can be used. Examples include *bancha* (*kukicha*) twig tea, and roasted grain teas. You may also drink a moderate amount of water (preferably spring or well water). Iced drinks are best avoided.

7. FOODS TO BE AVOIDED FOR BETTER HEALTH. Meat, eggs, animal fat, poultry, dairy products, including butter, yogurt, ice cream, milk, and cheese.
   Tropical or semi-tropical fruits and fruit juices, soda, artificial drinks and beverages, coffee, colored tea, and all aromatic, stimulant teas such as mint and peppermint tea.
   All artificially colored, preserved, sprayed, or chemically treated foods. All refined, polished grains, flours, and their derivatives. Mass-produced industrialized food including all canned and frozen foods.
   Hot spices, any aromatic, stimulant food or food accessory; artificial vinegar and other seasonings. Licit and illicit drugs are best avoided. (Medicines prescribed by a physician do not apply to this general guideline.) Alcohol and cigarettes should be kept to a minimum.

8. ADDITIONAL SUGGESTIONS. Cooking oil should be vegetable quality only. For optimum health, use only cold-pressed, mechanically expelled, unrefined sesame or corn oil in moderate amounts.
   Salt should be naturally processed sea salt and excessive use should be avoided. Traditional, non-chemicalized tamari soy sauce and miso may also be used like sea salt.
   You may eat regularly two to three times per day, as much as desired, provided the proportion is correct and chewing is thorough (at least 50 times per mouthful or until it becomes liquid). Please avoid eating for approximately three hours before sleeping.

A More Detailed Macrobiotic Food List

Items marked with an asterisk (*) are foods that may need to be avoided or restricted during the healing process. Look under the list of dietary modifications for specific problems for more information.

Grains:

Regular use	*Occasional use*	*Occasional flour products*
Short-grain brown rice	Long-grain brown rice	Whole wheat noodles*
Medium-grain brown rice	Sweet brown rice	*Udon* noodles*
Barley	*Mochi*	*Somen* noodles*
Pearl barley	Cracked wheat, bulgur	*Soba* noodles (buckwheat)*
Millet	Steel cut oats	Unyeasted whole wheat bread*
Corn	Rolled oats*	Unyeasted rye bread*
Corn on the cob	Corn grits*	*Fu**
Whole oats	Cornmeal*	*Seitan**
Wheat berries	Rye flakes	
Buckwheat*	Couscous	
Rye		

Vegetables:

Regular use	*Occasional use*	*Avoid*
Acorn squash	Celery*	Artichoke
Bok choy	Chives*	Bamboo shoots
Broccoli	Coltsfoot*	Beets
Brussels sprouts	Cucumber*	Curley dock
Burdock	Endive*	Eggplant
Butternut squash	Escarole*	Fennel
Cabbage	Green beans*	Ferns
Carrots & their tops	Green peas*	Ginseng
Cauliflower	Iceberg lettuce*	Green & red peppers
Chinese cabbage	Jerusalem artichoke*	New Zealand spinach
Collard greens	Kohlrabi*	Okra
Daikon & their tops	Lambsquarters*	Plantain
Dandelion roots, leaves	Mushrooms*	Purslane & shepard's purse
Hubbard squash	Patty pan squash*	Potato
Hokkaido pumpkin	Romaine lettuce*	Sorrel
Jinenjo	Salsify*	Spinach
Kale	*Shiitake* mushrooms*	Sweet potato
Leeks	Snap beans*	Swiss chard
Lotus root	Snow peas*	Tomato
Mustard greens	Sprouts*	Taro potato (albi)
Onion	Summer squash*	Yams
Parsley	Wax beans*	Zucchini
Parsnip		

Pumpkin
Radish
Red cabbage
Rutabaga
Scallions
Turnips & greens
Watercress

Beans:

Regular use	*Occasional use*	*Occasional bean substitutes*
Azuki beans	Black-eyed peas*	Dried *tofu*
Black soybeans	Black turtle beans*	Fresh tofu*
Chick-peas (garbanzos)	Great northern beans*	*Natto**
Lentils (green)	Kidney beans*	*Tempeh**
	Lima beans*	
	Mung Beans*	
	Navy beans*	
	Pinto beans*	
	Soybeans*	
	Split peas*	
	Whole dried peas*	

Sea Vegetables:

All these sea vegetables can be used regularly. *Arame*, *Hijiki*, Kombu, toasted *Nori*, Wakame, Dulse, Agar-agar, Irish moss, *Mekabu*.

Fruits (usually cooked or dried):

Occasional use	*Avoid*
Apples*	Avocados
Apricots*	Bananas
Blueberries*	Coconuts
Blackberries*	Dates
Cantaloupes*	Figs
Cherries*	Grapefruit
Grapes*	Kiwi fruit
Lemons (small amounts of juice for cooking)*	Oranges
	Mangoes
Peaches*	Papayas
Pears*	Persimmons
Plums*	Pineapple
Raisins*	All other tropical fruits
Raspberries*	

Strawberries*
Watermelon*

Seeds and Nuts:

Occasional use	*Avoid*
Almonds*	Brazil nuts
Chestnuts*	Caraway seeds
Peanuts*	Cashews
Pumpkin seeds*	Hazel nuts
Sesame seeds*	Macadamian nuts
Sunflower seeds*	Pistachios
Walnuts*	Poppy seeds
	Spanish peanuts
	All tropical nuts

Animal Foods and Their Products:

Occasional use	*Avoid*
Carp*	Red-meat fish
Clams*	Chicken
Cod*	All fowl
Flounder*	Eggs
Halibut*	All mammals
Lobster*	All dairy products
Oysters*	
Trout*	
Red snapper*	
Sole*	
White-meat fish in general*	

Pickles:

Regular use	*Avoid*
Bran pickles	Commercial dill pickles
Brine pickles	Herb pickles
Miso bran pickles	Garlic pickles
Miso pickles	Spiced pickles
Pressed pickles	Apple cider vinegar pickles
Sauerkraut	Wine vinegar pickles
Tamari pickles	
Takuan pickles	

Sweets:

Regular use	*Occasional use*	*Avoid*
Cabbage	*Amazaké* *	All tropical fruits

Carrots	Barley malt*	Brown sugar
Daikon	Chestnuts*	Carob
Onions	*See* fruit list*	Chocolate
Parsnips	Hot apple cider*	Fructose
Pumpkin	Hot apple juice*	Honey
Squash	Rice malt syrup*	Maple syrup
		Molasses
		White sugar

Beverages:

Regular use	*Occasional use*	*Infrequent use*	*Avoid*
Bancha twig tea (Kukicha)	Grain coffee (100% grain)	Green tea*	Distilled water
Bancha stem tea	Dandelion tea	Vegetable juices*	Coffee
Roasted barley tea	Kombu tea	Juices of fruits from fruit list*	Cold, iced drinks
Roasted brown rice tea	Umeboshi tea	Beer*	Hard liquor
Spring water	*Mu* tea	*Saké**	Herb teas
Well water			Mineral water & all bubbly water
			Regular tea
			Stimulants
			Sugared drinks
			Tap water
			Whiskey
			Wine

Seasonings and Oils:

Regular use	*Occasional use*	*Avoid*
Natural miso	Corn oil*	Animal fats
Dark sesame oil*	Ginger*	Butter & cream
Light sesame oil*	Horseradish*	Coconut oil
Natural soy sauce	*Mirin**	Cottonseed oil
Tamari soy sauce	Olive oil*	Commercial dressings
Unrefined white sea salt	Rice vinegar*	Garlic
Umeboshi plum & paste	Safflower oil*	Linseed oil
Umeboshi vinegar	Sunflower oil*	Margarine
		Mayonnaise
		Commercial miso
		Mustard
		Pepper
		Peanut oil
		Table salt
		All commercial seasonings

Soybean oil
Commercial soy sauce
All spices

Condiments:

Main condiments	*Other condiments*
Gomashio (sesame salt)	Brown rice vinegar
Sea vegetable powder	Cooked miso with scallions & onions
Sea vegetable powder with roasted sesame seeds	Nori condiment
Tekka	Roasted sesame seeds
Umeboshi plum	*Shiso* leaves & roasted sesame seeds
	Shio Kombu
	Umeboshi plum with raw scallions/onions
	Umeboshi vinegar

Snacks:

You can have leftovers, noodles, popcorn (unbuttered), puffed whole cereal grain, rice balls, rice cakes, roasted seeds, *sushi*, and whole wheat bread.

Cooking and Preparation Methods:

Regular use	*Occasional use*
Pressure-cooking	Sautéing*
Boiling	Stir-frying*
Steaming	Raw*
Waterless	Deep-frying*
Soup	*Tempura**
Pickling	Baking*
Oil-less sautéing (with water)	
Pressing	

Cooking Aspects to Change for Variety:

1. Selections of foods within the categories of grains, vegetables, beans, sea vegetables, and so on;
2. Methods of cooking;
3. Ways of cutting vegetables;
4. Amount of water used;
5. Amount and kind of seasoning and condiments used;
6. Length of cooking time;
7. Use of a higher or lower flame;
8. Varying the combination of foods and dishes;

9. Seasonal cooking adjustments.

Way of Life Suggestions and Reminders

- Maintain the dream and image of health, peace, and abundance for yourself, others and the world.
- Live each day happily without being preoccupied with your health, and stay mentally and physically alert and active.
- View everything and everyone you meet with gratitude. Offer thanks before and after each meal.
- It is best to retire before midnight and to get up early in the morning, especially with the sunrise.
- It is best to avoid wearing synthetic or woolen clothing directly against the skin. Wear cotton as much as possible, especially for undergarments. Avoid excessive metallic accessories on the fingers, wrists, or neck. Keep such ornaments simple and graceful.
- If your strength permits, go outdoors in simple clothing. Walk on the grass, beach, or soil up to one half hour every day.
- Keep your home (and other surroundings) in good order, from the kitchen, bathroom, bedroom, living room, to every corner of the house.
- Initiate and maintain an active correspondence, extending best wishes to your family and friends. Also maintain good relationships with everyone around you.
- Avoid taking long hot baths or showers unless you have been consuming too much salt or animal food.
- Scrub your entire body with a hot, damp towel until the skin becomes red, every morning or every night before retiring. If that is not possible, at least scrub your hands, feet, fingers and toes.
- Avoid chemically perfumed cosmetics. For care of the teeth, brush with natural preparations or sea salt.
- If your condition permits, exercise regularly as part of your daily life, including activities like scrubbing floors, cleaning windows, and so on, as well as exercise programs such as yoga, dance, sports, and martial arts.
- Avoid using electric cooking devices (ovens or ranges) or microwave ovens. Convert to a gas or wood stove at the earliest opportunity.
- It is best to minimize the frequent use of color television and computer display units.
- Include some large green plants in your house to freshen and enrich the oxygen content of the air in your home.

3. The Cause of Arthritis

Although its symptoms take many forms, arthritis can be classified into two distinct categories, according to cause:

- *Yin Arthritis*—produced by excessive intake of more extreme yin foods and beverages, such as fruits, fruit juice—especially tropical and semi-tropical varieties—spices, stimulant and aromatic herbs and beverages, soft drinks, sugar, artificial sweeteners, honey, chocolate, and vinegars, as well as excessive intake of tomato, eggplant, potato, and other vegetables of tropical origin.

- *Yang Arthritis*—caused by excessive intake of the more extreme yang food categories, including meat, eggs, shellfish, and other animal foods. Large amounts of salt and other minerals, including the excessive intake of calcium associated with the regular consumption of dairy foods, also creates a more yang arthritic condition.

Despite these differences, however, both types of arthritis are aggravated to varying degrees by the consumption of excessive oil and fat from either animal or vegetable sources. In addition, both types are accelerated by excessive intake of liquid and icy cold drinks such as soda, beer, and alcoholic drinks, and other cold beverages. Ice cream is of course one of the major contributing factors.

We can also classify the major types of arthritis according to the relative degree of more yin or yang energy they represent. Within the more yang category, for example, some varieties are more yang, or constrictive, and within the more yin category, certain varieties are moderately yin, or expansive, while others are more extreme. The traditional model of the five transformations, or energy changes, is an invaluable tool in further understanding the dietary and way of life causes of these conditions.

The five energies offer a more detailed explanation of the continual cycling between expansion and contraction, or yin and yang, that all things go through. The five stages of energy are illustrated in Figure 4.

The stages of upward and expanding energy are more yin; downward and condensed energy are more yang; while floating energy,

Fig. 4 The Five Stages of Energy

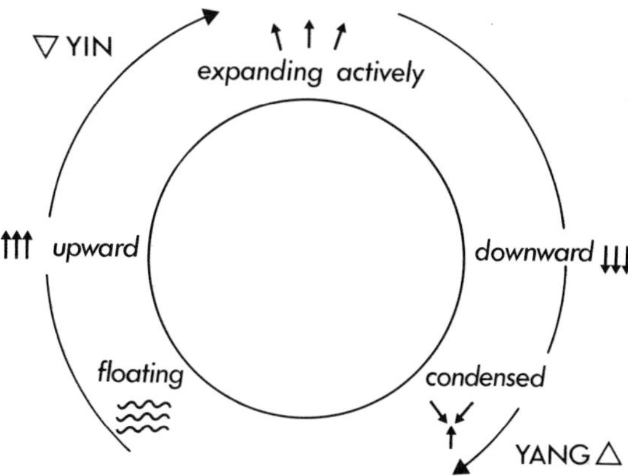

although at the bottom of the chart, is somewhat in between, and has characteristics of both tendencies.

As we saw earlier, the symptoms of arthritis can be divided into more yin and more yang categories, which also correlate to the five stages of energy:

More Yin Symptoms

- More generalized involvement of the body with a larger number of accompanying symptoms
- More inflammation
- More swelling
- More intense cyclic pain
- Involvement of more peripheral regions of the body

These symptoms are primarily more expansive in tendency. The stronger each of these is, and the more of them there are, the greater the degree of expansive energy the condition represents.

More Yang Symptoms

- Less general body involvement with fewer additional symptoms
- Less inflammation
- More chronic, deeper pain
- More central and lower-body involvement

The greater the extent to which these symptoms appear, the greater the degree of more yang energy the particular type of arthritis represents.

More than one hundred varieties of arthritis have been identified so far. However, they can all be classified into either more yin or more yang varieties (some represent extremes of both energies), and further, into five major categories according to the five transformations. Five major types of arthritis—*rheumatoid arthritis*, *osteoarthritis*, *lupus*, *ankylosing spondylitis*, and *gout*—can serve as examples in our classification, from which the other varieties can then be categorized. These five major types of arthritis are classified in the following chart and table:

Fig. 5 Five Types of Arthritis

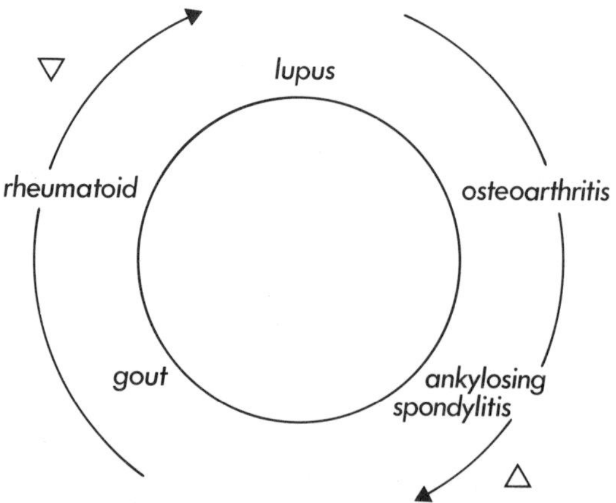

The cause of arthritis is rooted in our daily diet and way of life. The principle of yin and yang and the five stages of energy can help us to understand these causes, and enable us to orient our diet and way of life so as to avoid, and in many cases, recover from arthritis. In the following chapter, we discuss modifications in the standard macrobiotic diet that can help in serving this purpose.

On another level, arthritis can be seen as a form of premature aging. When they are healthy, children have soft and flexible joints and muscles. Their bodily flexidility is reflected in their mental condition: children are resilient, open minded, enthusiastic, and original. Life is filled with possibilities and adventure.

Arthritis represents the opposite condition, in which our body and mind are becoming progressively more rigid and inflexible.

Although the number of people with diagnosed arthritis is in the millions, the number of people with the beginning stages of body and joint hardening is actually much higher—in fact, the vast majority of people in the modern world experience this condition to one degree or another.

Type	*Primary Symptoms*	*Corresponding Energy*	*Major Food Causes* (when eaten excessively)
Rheumatoid arthritis	Swelling and inflammation of joint; intense cyclic pain that can become chronic; various accompanying symptoms	Excessive upward energy (more yin)	Fruits and fruit juices (especially tropical varieties such as banana, pineapple, citrus, and others); spices; concentrated sweeteners; alcohol; animal fats; including those in milk and poultry; tropical origin vegetables
Lupus	Joint pain and tenderness on motion (knuckles and wrists primarily affected, especially middle finger); many accompanying symptoms	Excessive expanding energy (more extreme yin)	Sugar and artificial sweeteners; tropical fruits; ice cream; chocolate; soft drinks; chemicals, drugs and medications; animal fats; tropical-origin vegetables
Osteoarthritis	Erosion of cartilage; narrowing of joint space; development of bony growths in joint; usually few or no accompanying symptoms	Excessive downward energy (more yang)	Animal fats, including those in meat, eggs, poultry, and dairy products; fruits; concentrated sweeteners; iced foods and drinks
Ankylosing Spondylitis	Inflammation where tendon or ligament attaches to bone, resulting in fusion of the joint (usually begins at lower spine and moves upward)	Excessive condensed energy (more extreme yang)	Meat, eggs, chicken, hard salty cheese; salt and other minerals; baked flour products; milk; butter
Gout	Swelling, inflammation, and pain in joints, especially at the base of the large toe; pain occurs mostly at night and is cyclic	Excessive floating energy (extreme yin and yang combined)	Extreme combinations, such as plenty of meat and alcohol; cheese and wine; rich sugary desserts; heavy sauces and gravies; chilled or iced foods or beverages

To test yourself for this condition—which we may refer to as *pre-arthritis*—place your hands together as in the above diagram. If you cannot push your fingers to a 90-degree angle, you are already experiencing inflexibility and hardening of the joints.

Fig. 6 Test for Joint Flexibility

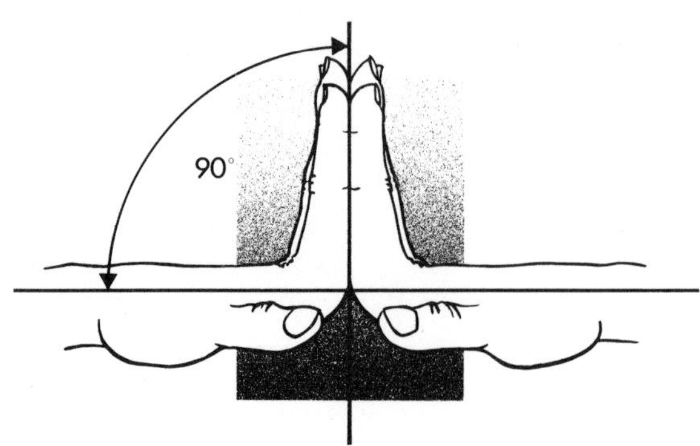

This condition often begins in childhood when we consume the modern diet high in animal foods—including meat, chicken, butter, milk, eggs, and cheese, together with tropical fruit juices, sugar, soft drinks, and ice cream. Hardening of the arteries due to the buildup of fat and cholesterol, is related to hardening of the joints, and muscles. Today, this condition also begins in youth, and researchers have begun to see fatty streaks in the arteries of elementary school children.

If we eat according to the natural order, there is no reason why we cannot enjoy physical and mental flexibility throughout life. The macrobiotic way of eating is the key to avoiding arthritis and maintaining a free and flexible life.

4. Dietary Adjustments for Arthritis

In Chapter 2, we looked at the Standard Macrobiotic Diet in general. By itself, this is enough to prevent many cases of arthritis from developing, and can serve as the foundation for continuing health. However, in cases where arthritis already exists, it is necessary to make some additional adjustments in this general dietary plan, to be followed for several months or until the condition improves, after which, the more general standard dietary approach may be adopted.

Both yin and yang varieties of arthritis reflect a basic extremism or imbalance in the body as a whole; so it is important in either case to avoid overly one-sided eating. Try to present a balanced mix of both more yin and more yang energies at each meal, and try to cultivate a keen sense of balance in the aesthetic aspects of your cooking, such as complementing contrasting colors, textures, and tastes.

General Recommendations for Arthritis

1. Extreme categories of both yin and yang foods are best avoided; in general, stay within the guidelines of the Standard Macrobiotic Diet. It is preferable to eat cooked foods only, although up to one-third of your vegetables may be lightly or quickly cooked. The consumption of both animal food and fruit is best kept to a minimum, and the use of salt, miso, tamari soy sauce and other salty seasonings or condiments is best kept moderate.

2. When selecting vegetables, it is advisable to avoid potatoes, tomatoes, eggplant, spinach, asparagus, avocados, beets, zucchini, and mushrooms (with the exception of shiitake mushrooms). The main food in the daily diet can be whole grains, while supplemental foods may include cooked vegetables, beans, sea vegetables, and if desired, small portions of animal food such as fish and seafood, and an occasional small volume of cooked or dried fruit.

3. As a special therapeutic dish, cook dried, shredded daikon with kombu and light tamari soy sauce to taste. Miso and scallions

cooked together with several drops of sesame oil is also beneficial when used occasionally as a condiment.

4. The use of wild vegetables such as fresh dandelion, watercress, and others can also be helpful. Prepare them by first sautéing with a small amount of sesame oil, then adding a little water and simmering.

5. Arthritis is commonly accompanied by chronic intestinal disorders. Thorough chewing of food is therefore essential, preferably 80 to 100 times or more per mouthful, until the food becomes completely liquified.

6. It is important for persons with arthritis to have regular, daily bowel movements. If they experience constipation, dishes such as kanten, boiled salad, steamed greens, or vegetables sautéed in a small amount of sesame oil can be eaten. If constipation persists, a mild salt-water or salt-bancha enema can be given.

7. A hot body scrub using a medium-sized towel dipped in plain hot water can be done twice per day. Begin with the hands and fingers, and work your way to the arms, shoulders, neck and head, back, abdomen, buttocks, and so on, finishing with the feet and toes. Reheat the towel before you do each section of the body, and scrub until the skin becomes slightly red or the circulation becomes active.

   Part of the problem of arthritis is due to accumulation of excess fat—mostly from animal sources and simple sugars—and minerals in and around the joints. These accumulations are accelerated when a thin layer of fat builds up under the skin, again, due largely to the chronic overconsumption of animal fats. The excessive factors normally discharged through the skin are thus blocked and held within the body. Daily body scrubbing helps activate circulation and the break down of these accumulations.

8. In severe cases, where the person is experiencing tightness or inflexibility, you may scrub the body with a hot ginger towel instead of using plain hot water. This may be done daily for some period in more severe cases, or several times per week in less severe cases.

9. Hot-towel compresses may be applied daily to joints or hardened body parts to relieve pain and dissolve stagnation, except in cases of active inflammation or swelling. Hot ginger towels

(ginger compresses) may be used in more severe cases. It is also helpful in more severe cases to soak swollen fingers and hands, or both feet in hot ginger water for about ten minutes.

10. Another helpful external treatment for arthritic persons is the periodic application of a ginger compress on the abdominal area. This can be done several times per week or more often in severe cases. Of course, as with all dietary and home applications, it is recommended that advice be sought from a qualified macrobiotic teacher or center. A further recommendation is to rub down along the spine with a towel dipped in hot ginger water. (This can be especially helpful in cases of ankylosing spondylitis.) Soak a towel in the water, squeeze, and then rub the area until it becomes red.

Below are general recommendations for the five major types of arthritis, based on the understanding of their yin or yang causes. For more yang types of arthritis (ie: osteoarthritis, ankylosing spondylitis, and gout) slightly more yin energies are emphasized in the selection and preparation of daily foods. For more yin forms of arthritis, including conditions such as rheumatoid arthritis and lupus, slightly more yang energies are emphasized. It bears repeating, though, that all conditions still need both energies, and it is important not to be one-sided in your cooking and selection of foods.

Dietary Recommendations for the Five Major Types of Arthritis

In the following section, each of the five major types of arthritis are listed with appropriate dietary suggestions. These guidelines provide the reader with a direct dietary outline to be used in their recovery of health. The effectiveness of these suggestions, that is, to what degree arthritic conditions can be changed, is based on the individual's skill in cooking the recommended foods, and on lifestyle practices such as chewing thoroughly. In order to maximize an individual's opportunity for recovery, it is recommended that the companion book on arthritis, in the *Macrobiotic Health Education Series.* be consulted. This book contains clear, simple explanations that include the proper selection of foods, easy to follow lifestyle guidelines, and the macrobiotic view of the cause of arthritis.

In addition, we recommend that all persons seeking to implement macrobiotic dietary guidelines contact a macrobiotic center for advice. The guidelines presented below, for example, can be generally observed for several months, at which time, adjustments may be required. Also, these guidelines are not substitutes for medical advice. Persons with serious conditions are advised to contact the appropriate medical or nutritional professional in addition to macrobiotic practice.

Dietary Suggestions for Rheumatoid Arthritis:

Cooking Methods: Pressure-cooking, boiling, nishime, kinpira, and water sautéing can be emphasized while other methods can be used more occasionally.

Whole Grains: Short-grain brown rice can be eaten daily, and should become the primary grain. It can be cooked with a pinch of sea salt or half-inch piece of kombu sea vegetable per cup of rice. Brown rice can also be eaten in combination with other grains and smaller types of beans. Secondary grains can include millet, whole wheat berries, barley, and others. Whole wheat noodles, called udon, can be eaten several times per week in soup.

It is best for the time being to avoid frequent intake of baked flour products such as cookies, crackers, chips, and the like, although high-quality unyeasted sourdough bread can be eaten several times per week. Breakfast porridge, made by adding water to leftover whole grains and cooking for a short time, can be eaten daily, however oatmeal made from rolled or steel-cut oats is best avoided temporarily. Whole oats are best. Soft brown rice (*kayu*) is an ideal breakfast cereal.

Soups: One cup or bowl of miso soup can be taken daily, preferably using either *mugi* (barley) or *Hatcho* (soybean) miso. This soup can include sea vegetables, either wakame or kombu, and a variety of vegetables, especially daikon, leafy greens, and sweet-tasting vegetables. A mild-tasting soup is preferable for daily use. A second cup or bowl of soup composed of different ingredients such as whole grains or beans may be taken for variety during the course of the day. It is important to use sea vegetables when preparing soups.

Vegetables: All three types of vegetables—leafy, round, and root—can be consumed daily, using a variety of cooking styles. However, daikon roots and leaves are especially helpful for this condition and should be included on a regular basis. For the first month, it is best not to use oil in cooking. During the second month, oil can be used in sautéing about once per week, and during the third month, about twice per week. Raw salads are best not taken until the symptoms of arthritis diminish somewhat; however boiled and pressed salads can be eaten daily or every other day. Kinpira (burdock and carrot dish) and nishime-style vegetables are helpful for this condition and can be eaten several times per week. Contracted leafy greens (daikon, turnip, carrot, etc.) are also helpful.

Beans and Bean Products: Smaller beans (azuki, chick-pea, lentil, and black soybeans) can be taken daily, about one-half-cup serving size. Larger beans are best not eaten for the first month, during the second month they can be taken two or three times per month. Tempeh and dried tofu can be eaten every other day in a variety of dishes. Fresh tofu can be used in small amounts once or twice per week.

Sea Vegetables: Wakame and kombu are used daily in soup, with vegetables, and with beans. Arame and hijiki side dishes can be eaten two or three times per week, and a sheet of toasted nori can be consumed daily. Sea vegetables can be used daily in moderate amounts.

Condiments: Condiments such as gomashio and sea-vegetable powders can be used in small volume on a rotating daily basis. Gomashio can be made in a 16 to 1 proportion of sesame seeds to sea salt. Umeboshi plums can be eaten two or three times per week. Roasted shiso leaves and nori condiment are helpful supplementary condiments, and can be eaten two or three times per week, as can tekka. It is best to avoid umeboshi vinegar or brown rice vinegar during episodes of joint pain.

Pickles: A small volume of naturally fermented pickles or sauerkraut can be eaten each day. Pickles with a strong sour taste are best minimized until the condition improves. If pickles have an excessively salty flavor, rinse them briefly under cold water before eating. Pickled daikon, known as takuan, can be helpful when eaten several times per week. Several small slices at a time are enough.

Fish and Seafood: It is best to use white-meat fish only, about once or twice per week if desired. Fish can be steamed, broiled, or cooked in soup. Fish and seafood are best eaten with a garnish of grated raw daikon or carrot.

Fruit: With swelling and inflammation, raw fruit or fruit juice is best minimized. A small, dessert-sized portion of cooked northern varieties of fruit can be eaten several times per week if desired. Dried fruit such as raisins or apples can occasionally be used in small amounts for sweetness. Among northern fruits, cooked or dried peaches are especially helpful and can be used most often. A small volume of fresh peaches can be eaten with a pinch of sea salt in summer.

Nuts: It is best to limit the intake of nuts and nut butters until the condition improves. Dried chestnuts can occasionally be cooked with rice, sweet rice, or azuki beans for a sweet flavor.

Seeds: A small volume of lightly roasted sesame, pumpkin, or squash seeds can be eaten. Sunflower seeds are best avoided temporarily or taken only in summer in small volume.

Snacks: A moderate amount of snacks such as popcorn, rice cakes, and puffed cereals can be eaten. Sushi, rice balls, left-overs, noodles, and occasional sourdough bread can also be eaten in moderate amounts as snacks.

Sweet Vegetables: Several varieties of sweet vegetables, such as carrots, squash, onions, and cabbage can be used daily in cooking.

Additional Sweets: Brown rice syrup is the most preferred concentrated grain sweetener for this condition. Several teaspoons per week can be added to breakfast cereal, tea, or used in making dessert.

Beverages: Beverages such as bancha tea, spring water, and grain teas may be consumed as thirst requires. Other suggested beverages can be taken on an occasional basis. A half cup of carrot juice, not icy cold, may be taken once or twice per week. However, if there is pain in the joints, it is best to wait on this drink.

Seasonings: Miso, tamari soy sauce, sea salt, and other seasonings are best used moderately in cooking. Seasonings that are more stimulating, such as ginger and horseradish, are best minimized for the time being.

Special Drinks: Sweet-vegetable broth can be taken, one cup daily (see chapter on *Beverages* for recipe). Ume-sho-kuzu can be taken twice per week for several weeks. Grated daikon (1/3 of a cup) plus grated carrot (1/3 of a cup) with water added to make one full cup can also be included several times per week for one month. These ingredients are simmered for two to three minutes with a few drops of tamari soy sauce. Roasted brown rice tea can be used alternately with bancha as a primary beverage for this condition.

Home Care: For swollen, hot joints, a plaster made of raw leafy greens mashed in a suribachi, or a tofu and greens plaster (mash equal proportions together in a suribachi) can be applied directly to the painful joint (see chapter on *Home Care*).

Lifestyle Suggestions: Use a hot, damp cloth to scrub the body daily, morning and evening before bed.
Chew very well, until food turns into liquid.
Do not take long baths or showers.
Rings, watches, and other jewelry and metallic accessories are best not worn, especially in areas where the joint is painful.

Dietary Suggestions for Lupus:

Cooking Methods: Nishime, kinpira, nitsuke, water sautéing, and boiling can be emphasized.

Whole Grains: Pressure-cooked short-grain brown rice can be eaten daily, by itself or in combination with other grains and smaller beans. Secondary grains such as barley, millet, and corn on the cob (when in season) can be prepared. Whole wheat noodles, called udon, can be eaten several times per week in broth. It is best for a time to avoid baked flour products, except for occasional sourdough, unyeasted bread. Buckwheat noodles, called soba, and whole grain buckwheat, called kasha, can be eaten once per week or so to help strengthen the condition.

Soup: One cup or bowl of miso soup can be taken daily, seasoned with the proper amount of mugi or *Hatcho* miso. Wakame or kombu, plus a good variety of vegetables, can also be used. A second cup or bowl of soup that includes a different combination of ingredients and seasonings can be enjoyed every day for variety.

Vegetables: A wide variety of vegetables can be eaten daily, using the full range of cooking styles. Burdock root is especially helpful for this condition and can be included several times per week. Raw salad is best avoided for a while, so boiled and pressed salads, or steamed greens, can be used daily. The use of oil in cooking can be avoided for about one month. During the second month, oil can be used once per week; during the third month, once or twice per week. Among special dishes, azuki beans cooked with squash and kombu; burdock and carrot kinpira; daikon, carrots, and turnips cooked with their green tops; dried, shredded daikon cooked with kombu; and nishime are especially helpful.

Beans and Bean Products: Smaller, low-fat beans (azuki, chick-pea, lentil, black soybeans) are preferred for daily use. The volume consumed can be up to a half cup per day. The larger, more fatty beans are best avoided for the first month. After this, they can be included once every ten days or so. Bean products like tempeh, tofu, and dried tofu can be included three or four times per week.

Sea Vegetables: Kombu and wakame can be used daily in soups, with vegetables, and in bean or other dishes. Hijiki or arame can be made in separate side dishes and included two or three times per week. A sheet of toasted nori can be consumed daily with rice balls or sushi, or as a garnish or snack.

Condiments: Gomashio and sea-vegetable powders can be used daily. Gomashio can be made in a 16 to 1 proportion of sesame seeds to sea salt. High-quality black sesame seeds are helpful if they can be obtained. Umeboshi plums can be used three or four times per week with whole grains or with tea. Two special condiments can be used several times per week: shio kombu and nori condiment. (Use one or two pieces of shio kombu or a teaspoon of nori condiment at a time.)

In cases of inflammation, it is best to minimize or avoid the use of brown rice vinegar and umeboshi vinegar until the condition improves. Tekka, a special condiment made from carrot, burdock, lotus root, and miso can be helpful when eaten with brown rice or other grains two or three times per week in very small amounts.

Pickles: A daily small volume of pickles can be taken after meals. If the taste is excessively salty, they can be briefly rinsed under cold water before eating. It is best to minimize or avoid very salty or very sour pickles.

Fish and Seafood: A small portion of white-meat fish can be prepared once or twice per week if necessary. If someone with lupus begins to feel very weak and lacks vitality, carp soup (*Koi-koku*) can be taken for several days (one cup or bowl per day), and then again one or two weeks later.

Fruit: If craved, a half cup of cooked northern fruit (with a pinch of sea salt) can be eaten several times per week. Raw fruits are best avoided until the condition improves. Dried chestnuts, when cooked with brown rice, sweet brown rice, or azuki beans are preferred over fruit. They can be eaten several times per week if desired.

Nuts: It is best not to eat nuts or nut butters until the condition improves and then only occasionally in small volume as snacks.

Seeds: A small volume of lightly roasted sesame, pumpkin, or squash seeds can be eaten as snacks. Sunflower seeds are best avoided until summer, and then eaten only on occasion in small quantities.

Snacks: Be careful not to eat too many dry snacks, such as rice cakes, popcorn, or puffed cereals, as these can cause a craving for liquid or sometimes sweets. Other snacks can be consumed moderately.

Sweet Vegetables: Sweet-tasting vegetables such as onions, squash, carrots, and cabbage can be used daily in cooking.

Additional Sweets: Minimize the use of concentrated sweeteners such as rice syrup or barley malt. If strongly craved, a small volume can be taken several times per week. Among concentrated natural sweeteners, the carbohydrate, or sugar, found in carrots can be especially helpful. Carrots can be simmered for a long time over a low flame to make carrot butter or carrot concentrate. Carrot butter can be used several times per week as a spread (on rice cakes or sourdough bread) or as a sweet condiment. Carrot concentrate can be dissolved in water and taken as a drink several times per week. Recipes for making these special foods are presented in the chapter on *Condiments*.

Beverages: Beverages such as bancha twig tea, grain teas, or grain coffee can be taken daily according to need. Carrot juice (about 1/2 cup) can be enjoyed several times per week, and if symptoms are active, it can be added later.

Seasonings: Seasonings are best used moderately. Seasonings that are more stimulating, such as ginger and horseradish, are best avoided until the condition improves.

Special Drinks: Sweet-vegetable broth can be taken, about one cup daily. Ume-sho-kuzu can be taken twice per week for about three weeks.

Home Care: A hot ginger compress or repeated hot towels (for 10 to 15 minutes) can be applied to the kidneys (middle back) and intestines (lower abdomen) to strengthen these organs in their function of eliminating excess. These compresses can be done about two or three times per week for about six weeks.

Lifestyle Suggestions: It is important to chew very well, until food becomes liquid in the mouth.
Every morning and evening before bed, a complete body scrub can be done with a cotton towel that is held under the hot faucet and wrung out.
One-half hour of daily walking is suggested as a comfortable form of exercise.
Do not take long hot baths or showers.
As often as possible, use organic quality grains, beans, and vegetables.

Dietary Suggestions for Osteoarthritis:

Cooking Methods: Quick boiling (ohitashi-style or boiled salad); steaming; quick sautéing (with or without oil), and pressing are helpful.

Whole Grains: Short-grain brown rice can be pressure-cooked with a pinch of sea salt and eaten daily. Brown rice can also be cooked in combination with other grains and smaller beans.

Barley, and especially pearl barley (hato mugi) can be especially helpful. It can be eaten two or three times per week with rice or in the form of soup. Secondary grains such as barley, millet, and corn on the cob (when in season) can be used.

It is best to limit the intake of baked flour products. If bread is craved, natural-quality sourdough (unyeasted) bread can be eaten several times per week, preferably steamed until soft. It is best to temporarily avoid rolled or steel-cut oats, as well as other cracked or flaked grains. If oats are craved, cook whole oats overnight on a very low flame. Noodles, preferably whole wheat noodles, called udon, can be eaten several times a week in broth.

Soup: One cup or bowl of miso soup can be taken daily with wakame, kombu, and a variety of vegetables, especially daikon, shiitake mushroom, and leafy greens. A variety of other soups can be used each day as a second cup or bowl. Soups are best when seasoned very lightly, avoiding a strong salty taste. Miso soup can be garnished with chopped scallions, chives, or parsley.

Vegetables: A wide range of vegetables can be eaten daily using a variety of combinations and cooking styles. Among vegetables, cooked dandelions are especially helpful and can be included two or three times per week (see chapter on *Vegetables*).

Raw salad is best avoided; however, the energy of boiled salad and steamed greens can be helpful, and these dishes can be included daily. The use of oil in cooking is best avoided for one month. During the second month, a small amount of sesame oil can be used several times per week. Occasional raw salad can be included once the condition improves.

Beans and Bean Products: Smaller beans (azuki, chick-pea, lentil, and black soybeans) are preferable for daily use. Bean products can be eaten daily or every other day. If someone is overweight, it is best to avoid larger beans for one month, after which they can be included once every week or ten days.

Sea vegetables: Kombu and wakame can be taken daily in soup, vegetables, and in bean dishes. Hijiki or arame can be prepared as side dishes two or three times per week. A sheet of toasted nori can be eaten daily.

Condiments: Gomashio, and sea-vegetable powders can be used daily. Gomashio can be made in a 16 to 1 proportion of sesame seeds to sea salt. Umeboshi plums, and brown rice or umeboshi vinegar can be eaten two or three times per week.

Pickles: A small volume of pickles may be eaten daily. If the taste is excessively salty, they can be briefly rinsed in cold water before eating. Quick, light pickles or sauerkraut are preferred for more regular use.

Fish: A small portion of white-meat fish can be eaten once or twice per week if desired. Shellfish and more fatty fish (ie: tuna, salmon, etc.) are best avoided. The fish can be prepared by either boiling, steaming, or in miso soup.

Fruit: Cooked northern fruits can be enjoyed as dessert about three times per week. Among these, plums are especially helpful and can be cooked in dessert from time to time. Raw fruit is best kept to a minimum until the condition improves.

Nuts: It is best to avoid nuts or nut butters until the condition improves, at which time they can be included from time to time as snacks.

Seeds: A small volume of lightly roasted sesame, pumpkin, or squash seeds can be eaten as snacks. Do not burn the seeds while roasting. Sunflower seeds are best avoided until summer, at which time they can be eaten in small quantities on occasion.

Snacks: Be careful not to eat too many dry snacks, such as rice cakes, popcorn, and puffed cereals. Other snacks can be consumed according to desire.

Sweet Vegetables: These can be used daily in cooking.

Additional Sweets: A small volume of barley malt (about one teaspoon) can be used several times per week on breakfast porridge, in dessert, or in tea. Other concentrated sweeteners can be used occasionally. Dried chestnuts may be cooked with brown rice or azuki beans from time to time as a sweet treat.

Beverages: Bancha twig tea, spring water, and grain teas can be taken daily. The volume depends on how thirsty a person is. Roasted barley tea (mugicha) or pearl-barley tea (hato mugicha) are especially helpful and can be alternated with bancha as main beverages.

Seasonings: Seasonings are best used moderately in daily cooking. Seasonings that are more stimulating, such as ginger and horseradish, are best avoided until the condition improves.

Special Drinks: Sweet-vegetable broth can be taken, about one cup daily for one month or longer if necessary. Then it can be taken two to three times per week. A drink made from grated daikon (1/3 of a cup), grated carrot (1/3 of a cup), and 1/3 of a cup of water can be taken two or three times per week for one month. Simmer for two or three minutes with a few drops of tamari soy sauce. Dandelion coffee, available at most natural food stores, is especially helpful for this condition. It can be used three or four times per week as a supplement to the other beverages for regular use.

Home Care: Hot towels or a hot ginger compress can be applied to painful joints whenever necessary to improve circulation and reduce hardening.

Lifestyle Suggestions: It is important to chew very well, until food becomes liquid in the mouth.
Every morning and evening before bed, a complete body scrud can be done with a hot cotton towel.
A half-hour daily walk is suggested as a form of comfortable exercise.
A short shower or bath can be taken daily.

Dietary Suggestions for Ankylosing Spondylitis:

Cooking Methods: Steaming, quick sautéing, ohitashi style boiling, quick pickling or pressing are helpful.

Whole Grains: Short-grain brown rice can be used daily, with medium-grain rice occasionally used as a supplement. Brown rice can also be cooked in combination with other grains and beans. It is best not to cook the grains until they become dry, so a little extra water can be used. Among the secondary grains, barley, and especially fresh corn can be helpful. Corn on the cob can be eaten often when it is available.

It is best for a time to minimize or avoid flour products such as cookies, crackers, muffins, and the like. Unyeasted sourdough bread—preferably steamed until soft—can be eaten several times per week. If oats are craved, whole oats can be cooked overnight over a very low flame and eaten for breakfast.

Whole wheat udon noodles can be eaten several times a week in light tamari broth. Buckwheat noodles and whole grain buckwheat are best avoided until the condition improves. Naturally processed corn grits can be used several times per week as a breakfast cereal.

Soup: One cup or bowl of miso soup, with wakame or kombu, and a variety of vegetables can be included daily. Summer greens, daikon, and shiitake mushrooms can be included in miso soup. A second bowl or cup of soup may also be included daily using a variety of other ingredients and seasonings. Corn and vegetable soup can be included several times per week. It is important to use a small piece of sea vegetable in preparing soup.

Vegetables: All three types of vegetables, leafy, root, and round, can be eaten daily, using a variety of combinations and cooking styles. Among the acceptable vegetables, cucumber is helpful to relax an overly tight condition. It can be served several times per week in salad and used to make pickles. The use of sesame oil in cooking is best kept to several times per week. Boiled salad and quickly steamed greens can be helpful when included daily.

Beans and Bean Products: The smaller beans (azuki, chick-peas, lentil, and black soybeans) and bean products can be used alternately on a daily basis. The volume consumed can average about half a cup daily. The larger beans are best taken about two or three times per month.

Sea Vegetables: Kombu and wakame can be eaten daily in soup, with vegetables, and in bean dishes. Hijiki or arame can be cooked as side dishes two or three times per week. A sheet of toasted nori can be eaten daily with rice balls, sushi, or as a garnish.

Condiments: Gomashio and sea-vegetable powders can be used daily. Gomashio can be made in a 16 to 1 proportion of sesame seeds to sea salt. Umeboshi plums can be eaten two or three times per week. However, it is best to minimize the use of brown rice vinegar and umeboshi vinegar if there is pain. Other condiments may be used several times per week.

Pickles: A small volume of pickles may be eaten daily. Quick, light pickles, including natural, non-spicy cucumber pickles, are preferred. If the taste is excessively salty, they can be briefly rinsed in cold water before eating.

Fish: A small portion of white-meat fish can be eaten once or twice per week. Other varieties of fish or shellfish are best avoided until the condition improves.

Fruit: Among fruits, apricots can be helpful for this condition. They, along with other cooked northern fruits can be enjoyed about three times per week on average. A small volume of dried apricots can be eaten on occasion, as can a small amount of fresh apricots.

Nuts: It is best to minimize or avoid nuts or nut butters until the condition improves.

Seeds: A small volume of lightly roasted sesame, pumpkin, or squash seeds can be eaten as snacks. It is important not to take a large amount of dry-roasted seeds. Sunflower seeds are best avoided until summer and then can be eaten in small quantities occasionally.

Snacks: A reduced volume of dry snacks such as rice cakes, popcorn, and puffed cereals is best. However, puffed whole corn can be helpful and can be used as a frequent snack. It can be eaten plain or together with amazake. Other snacks can be consumed moderately.

Sweet Vegetables: These can be used in daily cooking.

Additional Sweets: If extra sweetness is craved, a small volume of rice syrup, barley malt, or amazake can be included several times per week. Corn amazake can be especially good in this case. Dried chestnuts may also be cooked with grains or beans for added sweetness.

Beverages: Bancha tea, spring water, and grain teas can be taken daily. The amount depends upon how thirsty an individual may be. Carrot or apricot juice can be used once or twice per week if desired. All drinks should be warm or room temperature.

Seasonings: Seasonings are best used moderately in daily cooking. Seasonings that are more stimulating, such as ginger and horseradish, are best avoided for the time being.

Special Drinks: Sweet-vegetable broth can be taken two or three times per week. A drink made from grated carrot (1/3 of a cup), grated daikon (1/3 of a cup), and 1/3 of a cup of water can be taken several times per week, either raw or simmered. A few drops of tamari soy sauce can be added.

Home Care: Hot towels or a hot ginger compress can be applied to painful areas of the spine, especially when symptoms are present. Also, the whole spine can be rubbed vigorously with either of these hot compresses.

Lifestyle Suggestions: It is important to chew well, until food becomes liquid in the mouth.
Every morning and evening before bed, a complete body scrub can be done with a hot cotton cloth.
A daily short shower or bath can be taken.
If possible, a one-half-hour walk is suggested as a comfortable form of exercise.
Do not let yourself become cold, as this can cause tightness.

Special Suggestions
It is important to use sea salt, miso, and other seasonings in a moderate, balanced way so that food does not have an overly salty flavor.

Dietary Suggestions for Gout:

Cooking Methods: Boiling, nishime style, kinpira, long-sautéing, pressure-cooking, and nitsuke style are helpful.

Whole Grains: Short-grain brown rice can be the main grain for daily use. It can also be cooked with other grains and with azuki and other beans. Millet can be featured as a secondary grain, along with barley, fresh corn, and others.

It is best for a time to avoid baked flour products such as

cookies, muffins, and crackers, even those of natural, organic quality, until the condition improves. High-quality sourdough bread can be eaten several times per week.

If oats are craved, whole oats can be used as breakfast cereal. Whole wheat noodles, called udon, can be eaten several times a week in broth, while buckwheat is best avoided until the condition improves. Creamy, floury cereals or sauces are also best avoided.

Soup: One cup or bowl of miso soup can be included daily with wakame or kombu sea vegetable, and a variety of vegetables, especially daikon, shiitake mushroom, and leafy greens. A variety of other soups can be included, including millet and squash soup, purēed squash soup, and azuki bean soup.

Vegetables: Leafy, green, round, and root vegetables can be eaten daily, using a variety of combinations and cooking styles. Cabbage is especially helpful for this condition and can be served often, as can other sweet vegetables such as squash and onions. Raw salad is best minimized or avoided until the condition improves. The use of oil is best kept to a minimum. If swelling and pain are experienced, it may be necessary to avoid oil temporarily. Squash cooked with azuki beans and kombu can be helpful in providing additional sweetness and can be included two to four times per week.

Beans and Bean Products: Smaller beans (azuki, chick-peas, lentil, and black soybeans) can be used daily. The volume consumed can average about a half cup. Tempeh, tofu, dried tofu, and natto can also be included three or four times per week. If someone is overweight, it is best to avoid larger, fattier beans for about a month. Afterward, they can be used weekly.

Sea Vegetables: Kombu and wakame can be used daily in soups, with vegetables, and in bean dishes. Hijiki or arame can be included in side dishes two or three times per week. A sheet of toasted nori can be eaten daily.

Condiments: Gomashio and sea-vegetable powders can be used daily. Gomashio can be made in a 16 to 1 proportion of sesame seeds to sea salt. Umeboshi plums can be eaten two or three times per week. Other condiments may be used several times per week for variety. However, it is best to minimize the use of brown rice vinegar and umeboshi vinegar, especially when there is joint pain.

Pickles: A small volume of pickles can be eaten daily. If the taste is excessively salty, they can be briefly rinsed in cold water before eating.

Fish: Excessive consumption of animal protein and fat contributes to this condition. Therefore, it is best to eat a small proportion of white-meat fish only once or twice per week if craved. Fish can be eaten along with several tablespoons of grated daikon as garnish. Other varieties of seafood are best avoided until the condition improves.

Fruit: Cooked northern fruit can be eaten about three times a week as a dessert. Raw or dried fruits can be eaten occasionally in small volume if desired. Although not usually recommended in a temperate climate, the occasional use of dates in cooking can help stabilize this condition. Dates can be used to sweeten the azuki bean/chestnut dish mentioned previously. This dish can be taken about once per week for up to about six weeks. Please refer to the chapter on *Beans and Bean Products* for the recipe.

Sweet Vegetables: These can be used daily in cooking.

Additional Sweets: A small volume of concentrated sweeteners can be used once or twice a week if desired. Amazake can also be used on occasion.

Beverages: Bancha tea, spring water, and grain teas can be used daily. Carrot juice can be enjoyed several times per week if desired. It is important to avoid icy cold beverages and to not drink excessively.

Seasonings: Seasonings are best used moderately. Seasonings that are more stimulating, such as ginger or horseradish, are best avoided until the condition improves.

Special Drinks: Sweet-vegetable broth can be included two or three times per week, a cup at a time.

A drink made of grated carrot (1/3 of a cup), grated daikon (1/3 of a cup), and water (1/3 of a cup) can be taken two to three times per week for one month. Simmer this mixture over a low flame for two or three minutes and add tamari soy sauce. Kombu tea can also be taken several times per week until the condition improves.

Home Care: For pain in the joints, a tofu and raw greens plaster (half and half mashed in a suribachi) can be applied directly to the painful area. Raw greens or tofu can also be applied separately. These can be applied when the joint is painful, or two to three times per week for a month. A hot ginger compress can be applied to the kidney region twice a week for one month.

Lifestyle Suggestions: It is important to chew very well, until the food becomes liquid in the mouth.
Every morning and evening before bed, a complete body scrub can be done with a hot cotton towel.
A half-hour daily walk is suggested as a comfortable form of exercise.
A daily short shower or bath can be taken.
It is best not to smoke.
If the large toe area is afflicted, which happens in most cases of gout, it is important to wear cotton socks.

5. Menu Planning

When planning a menu, there are several things to consider.

1. The relative proportion of grains, vegetables, soup, beans, and so on in a meal as recommended in the Standard Macrobiotic Diet.

2. Adjustments for the individual types of arthritis (see *Dietary Adjustments for Arthritis* chapter).

3. Variety in meals. For instance, last night's dinner rice can be this morning's soft rice. It is most important, however, to have fresh soup and fresh, quickly boiled or blanched leafy greens every day. Therefore, boil only as many greens as are needed for one meal. To ensure variety, be sure to consider:

   A. *The types of vegetables and grains used.* Every day have some kind of root vegetable, fresh and leafy greens and, in some form, a small amount of sea vegetable. It is helpful to have brown rice every day, but there are many ways to vary this basic dish as you will see in the menu examples.
   B. *The seasonings, condiments, and pickles used.* (It is preferred that one has a small amount of pickles daily.)
   C. *The cooking methods employed.* Every day, have some quickly boiled or blanched greens, as well as pressure-cooked or longer-time cooked items.
   D. *The sizes, shapes, colors, and textures from dish to dish.* Use attractive garnishes to brighten your meals.

4. *Seasonal and climatic adjustments.* For hot weather, emphasize more fresh, lightly boiled or steamed vegetables, salads, less cooking time, and less oil and salt. For colder weather, emphasize more hearty, rich dishes, stews and thick soups, protein such as found in beans, root vegetables, and a little more salt and oil.

5. *Adjustments for the time of day.* Beans, hardy dishes, and stronger seasonings are best eaten for dinner. It is recommended that lunches and breakfasts be kept simple and light, otherwise one may feel heavy and sluggish throughout the day. Soft porridges and whole-grain cereals are delicious for breakfast.

6. *Adjustments for age.* For babies, younger children, and elderly

persons, serve more soft foods and sweet-tasting vegetables with a minimum amount of seasonings. It is preferred that babies do not eat any salt at all. Teens and adults can have more seasonings and more crisp, solid vegetables.

7. *Life-style adjustments.* People doing more physical exercise, work, and activities need more protein and hardy, rich dishes than do those who are more sedentary.

8. *Use as much of your leftovers as possible.* The menus below disregard leftovers to emphasize variety. Normally, a grain or bean dish, for example, can last for several days or more. Besides simply reheating leftovers, you can rework them into a new format; for instance, last night's dinner rice can be this morning's soft rice. Or you might want to add a few pieces of tofu when heating up yesterday's root vegetables. The possibilities are endless. All this adds more appeal and variety to your meals. It is most important, however, to have fresh, quickly boiled or blanched leafy greens every day. Therefore, boil only as many greens as you can have in one meal.

A General Seven Day Menu for all Types of Arthritis:

	BREAKFAST	LUNCH	DINNER
1.	Soft rice w/umeboshi Steamed greens Pickled Chinese cabbage Tea	Fu & vegetables Watercress sushi Tea	Pressure-cooked rice Clear soup Azuki/kombu/squash Kinpira carrot & burdock Boiled salad w/ume dressing Arame w/corn Apricot couscous cake Tea
2.	Miso soup w/tofu Rice balls Tea	Pressure-cooked millet & vegetables Boiled broccoli Tempeh & vegetables Tea	Gomoku Pureed carrot soup Nori condiment Corn on the cob Apple sauce Tea
3.	Soft millet w/shiso-green nori condiment Rutabaga/tamari pickle Broiled tofu Tea	Steamed leftover rice Scrambled tofu Boiled salad Tea	Pressure-cooked rice w/wheat berries Watercress tamari broth soup Chick-peas w/carrots & kombu Steamed greens Pickle

			Hijiki w/carrots & onions Tea
4.	Soft barley Red radish pickle Tea	Sushi Sautéed vegetables & tempeh Tea	Pressure-cooked millet w/corn Seitan & onions Boiled salad Shio kombu Cream of broccoli soup Stewed fruit w/kuzu Tea
5.	Miso soup Mochi Toasted nori Grated daikon Tea	Fried udon & vegetables Boiled watercress Tea	Pressure-cooked rice w/ barley Pureed squash soup Kombu carrot rolls Steamed greens Black soybeans Pickle Tea
6.	Soft whole oats Dulse/sesame condiment Onion/tamari pickle Tea	Ohagi (sesame & chestnut) Steamed greens Sautéed carrots Tea	Boiled rice Lentil soup Steamed mustard greens Pressed salad Sautéed vegetables Kanten
7.	Soft sweet rice & chestnuts Pickled daikon Tea	Udon & broth Boiled salad Tofu dressing Tea	Fried Rice & vegetables Miso soup Steamed fish Grated daikon Steamed greens Wakame/cucumber salad Tea

6. Cookware

Along with stocking good food, a kitchen needs to be equipped with a collection of essential cookware. Having the right tools at hand frees the mind to work with a more relaxed and creative attitude. This naturally has a profound effect on personal well-being as well as affecting the quality, taste, and appeal of meals. Also, some types of kitchen equipment should best be avoided as they may be detrimental to health, while others are a must for their beneficial influences. Listed below is a checklist of recommended kitchen equipment.

1. We recommend a gas stove as opposed to an electric one. There are several reasons for this:

   A. Electricity dissipates the molecular structure and strength of food by causing the electrons to bounce out of the atomic field, leaving the atom very unstable. Gas, on the other hand, just bounces the molecules around, while leaving them intact.

   B. It is very hard to fine-tune cooking with electricity. It is a conductive heat which first warms the coils and then the pot and its contents from the bottom up. The temperature cannot be changed quickly when turning to high or low because it takes some time to cool or heat the pot. Electricity makes it difficult to cook uniformly and it is possible that ingredients at the bottom of the pan can burn while those at the top need more cooking. A gas flame heats the surrounding air. Food thus cooks much more evenly, and the temperature can be adjusted immediately (a pot of water will instantly stop boiling the moment the flame is turned off, for example). Meals are more well cooked.

   C. Because of these drawbacks in electric cooking, a person may not feel satisfied with the meal and may crave strong salt or animal food (to counter the yin and weakening effects) which in turn causes a craving for excessive sweets and other yin foods. In other words, it becomes more of a struggle to eat in a balanced manner and thus to stay on the macrobiotic diet.

   A microwave oven should be avoided, particularly if a family member is sick. These ovens zap food with radioactive waves at three-billion-cycles per second (an electric stove runs at 60-cycles per second and actually generates a low form of radiation). It disintegrates instead of cooks food, and can cause the same effect in our body. Microwave cooking cannot help in regaining health, and it is suspected to contribute to certain types of illnesses.

After gas, wood is the best source of heat (followed by coal or charcoal) though it is impractical for most modern homes. It has a peaceful energy and at the same time it gives great strength to our foods.

2. Several stainless-steel pots of varying sizes. The steel does not interfere with the energies of the food. It is best to avoid aluminum because it is a poisonous substance and under high temperatures or when cooking very acidic (sweet) or alkaline (salty) foods, harmful toxins are released and mixed in with your ingredients.

   Cookware made out of glass (like Pyrex), earthenware, and enamelware are also excellent materials to cook in. (Be careful that you do not pour cold water into a heated enamel pot or leave it empty over a flame as this will cause it to crack. Let it cool off before washing it. It is also easily scratched so do not clean it with a steel-wool scrubber and use a wooden spoon when handling food inside it.)

3. At least one pressure cooker (stainless or enamel steel). This is an ideal pot for cooking grains, beans, root vegetables (like big chunks of burdock), squash, or anything that takes a long time to soften. The nutrients are better retained and everything is cooked more thoroughly, quickly, and with more energy than when prepared in a regular pot.

Fig. 7 Pressure Cooker

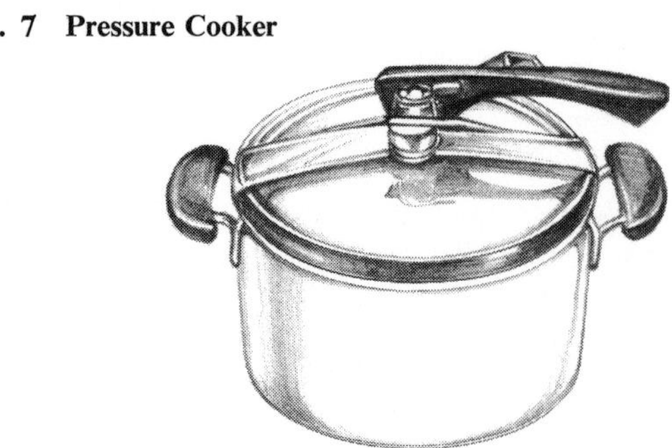

To use, put ingredients inside (not more than ¾ full), cover (don't forget to put the weight attachment on top), and over a medium-high flame, bring to pressure. You can tell the pressure is up when there is a lot of hissing and the weight begins to jiggle and shake. Then, immediately turn down the flame and, if needed, place a heat deflector underneath. Simmer (anywhere from 5 to 10 minutes to an hour or more depending on what is inside) until the food is done. Take the pot off the stove and let the pressure come down. You can let it come down naturally or rinse the pot under cold running water in the sink. This brings it down right away.

Before you cook, carefully take a good look at the cover. Inspect the hole (on which you place the weight) and make sure that it is not clogged. Otherwise, an explosion can occur when the pressure is high. Also, look at the rubber rings on the inside of the lid and in the pot itself where the rings touch. Remove any bits of food or other substances which may be stuck there as they will create a gap where steam can escape and as a result, the pressure will never build up.

4. Several cast-iron skillets for roasting and sautéing. Season them before their first use and from time to time thereafter. To do this, wash and dry them thoroughly. Then rub sesame oil all over (outside also) with a paper towel. The inside can be coated by rotating and tilting the pan over a flame. Place oiled pans in the oven at 225° to 250° F. for two to three hours. Then, let them sit for a few hours until they cool. Seasoning prevents the pans from rusting. For the same reason, do not soak cast-iron pans in hot, soapy water, and dry them thoroughly over a low flame after washing them.

5. One deep cast-iron pot for deep-frying. Cast iron is the best material to hold the intense heat of the oil.

6. Baking containers including pie plates, bread pans, muffin tins and so on. Again, avoid aluminum.

7. An optional *wok* (a Chinese-style skillet). The cast-iron skillets can effectively cover sautéing needs but a wok is great for light, and fast-cooking vegetables and fish.

8. Several stainless-steel mixing bowls in different sizes for washing and mixing food.

9. Large wooden serving bowls for grains. Wood allows the cooked grains to breathe. It also retards spoilage by absorbing any

excess water. The bowls need to be oiled periodically to prevent them from cracking. Heat some sesame oil, pour it into a completely dry bowl which is rotated until the inside is thoroughly oiled. Oil the outside also, with a brush or paper towel. Let it sit for a few hours until it dries completely.

10. Various other attractive serving containers made of glass, china, or ceramics. (Plastic is to be avoided.)
11. A stainless-steel or bamboo steamer.
12. A colander for rinsing noodles and other foods.
13. A fine-mesh strainer for washing seeds and grains.
14. A *suribachi* and pestle for making gomashio and other condiments. This is a Japanese ceramic bowl with grooves, made for crushing roasted sesame seeds, sea vegetables and so on.

Fig. 8 Suribachi and Pestle

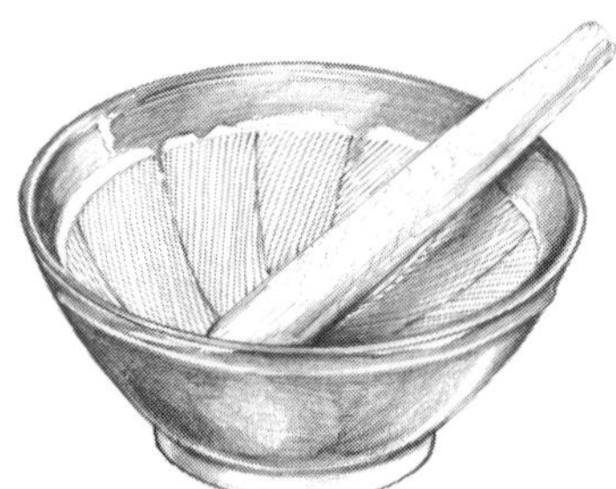

15. A food mill for pureeing cooked grains and vegetables. (An electric blender is more disruptive to the energies of foods. Instead of using one on a regular basis, save it for parties or special occasions when working with large volumes.)
16. A grain mill for grinding grains and nuts into flour. Flour is best when used soon after grinding. After being cracked, grain immediately starts to oxidize, and begins to lose some of its nutrients. Also, it is most delicious when fresh. (A local natural food store may have a good supply of flour as well.)
17. A pickle press for making pickles and pressed salads.
18. An earthenware crock with a wide mouth is good for making bran pickles, among other things.
19. Tea pot or kettle. Avoid aluminum.

20. A tea strainer for straining out leaves and twigs when serving the tea. A bamboo strainer, found in natural food and Oriental stores, is the best one to use.
21. Large glass jars for storing grains, beans, nuts, seeds, and other foods, as well as for making pickles.
22. Wooden cutting boards. Keep a separate one for fish and animal foods as their bacteria can have a toxic effect on vegetables.
23. Knives. The square-shaped Oriental knives are the easiest and the most efficient. They come in:
    A. carbon (which has a good sharp edge but rusts and chips easily),
    B. stainless steel (which does not rust but is not as sharp), and
    C. high-grade carbon with stainless steel which does not rust and is sharp as well (but is more expensive).

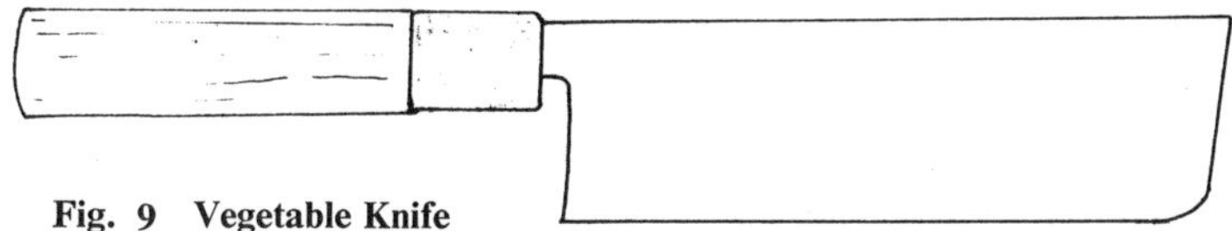

Fig. 9 Vegetable Knife

To protect the carbon knives, as soon as they are used, wash them in warm, soapy water, and then dry them immediately. If rust starts to appear, scrape it off with a steel-wool scrubber. Along with keeping knives as dry as possible, coating them with a little sesame oil after use will provide additional protection.

A sharpening stone will be needed to keep the edges of knifes sharp. Oil the stone with a vegetable oil or rinse it in water before use. Tilt the knife at a twenty-degree angle and sweep the blade against the stone in several circular motions. Use one hand to press down on the blade while the other hand holds the knife and moves it in circles. Sharpen the entire length of the edge. For more control, sharpen just one side (the right side for right handers and the left side for lefties). Do not use this knife for bread as its blade may be destroyed.

24. A bread knife. The best knife for cutting bread has a long, thin blade with a serrated edge.
25. A grater, most often used in macrobiotic cooking for grating fresh ginger, daikon, ca·rots, onions, lotus root, jinenjo, and taro potato.

26. A vegetable peeler, good for removing skins of cucumbers, apples and so on, when necessary.

27. A flame or heat deflector. This thin metal plate is placed underneath the pot or pressure cooker to even the flame and to help prevent the food from burning. Do not use the white asbestos deflectors as asbestos is poisonous.

28. An oil skimmer for lifting small bits of batter and food from tempura oil as well as for lifting vegetables from a pot of water.

29. A natural-bristle brush for brushing oil into skillets, cookie sheets, muffin tins, pie plates, and so on. Any small, clean, unused brush can be used.

30. Drop tops. These tops fit inside the pot and sit right on top of the food being cooked. This is an especially effective way to cook beans. Drop tops add some pressure but let steam escape and thus the food is cooked more thoroughly and softens more quickly.

31. Drop tops for pickles made in a keg such as bran pickles. A wooden one is best. A heavy stone or weight is placed on top for pressure. A plate is a good substitute if a wooden top cannot be found.

32. Vegetable brushes with natural bristles are best for washing vegetables. They can be found in natural or Oriental food stores.

33. Wooden spoons for stirring, mixing, scooping, and serving food before and after cooking. Wood has the best energy in interaction with food and is gentler to pots, pans, and bowls. Wooden spoons do not scratch cookware.

34. A bamboo rice paddle for handling and serving your grains.

Fig. 10 Rice Paddle

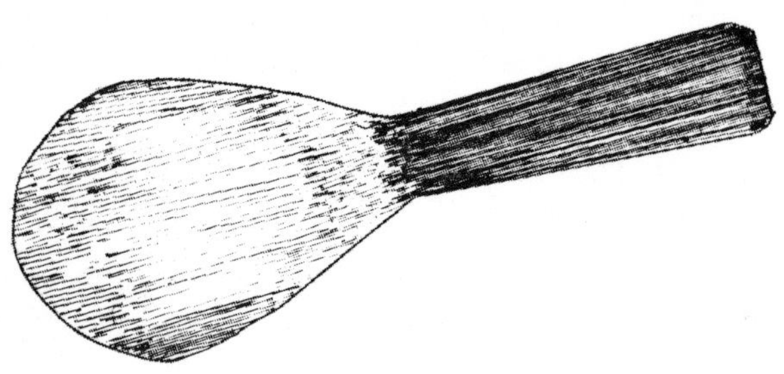

35. Soup ladles.
36. Rubber spatula for scraping batter, puréed food and so on from clean bowls.
37. A metal spatula for turning food over.
38. Cooking chopsticks. These are longer than the table version.
39. A rolling pin.
40. Measuring cups and spoons.
41. Sushi mats for making sushi and for covering cooked food. (They let air circulate and help retard spoilage.)
42. Bamboo mats. Also for covering food.
43. One hundred percent cotton cheesecloths, used as a cover when making pickles and also for making little sacks to contain foods in cooking (sort of like a tea bag).
44. Paper towels.

7. Cooking Attitude

Besides having good-quality food and proper cookware, to be a good cook, the right attitude and frame of mind are also necessary. Here is another check list.

1. A cook should leave all worries, problems, and angers behind as he or she relaxes mind and body into a peaceful, calm state of being. A cook's thoughts and emotions are mixed into the food and have an effect on anyone who eats it. Here are some things, among others, to remember while cooking.

   A. Pour love and healing vibrations into the food, and imagine that whoever eats it will become healthier and happier.

   B. Imagine that the food has the power to help individuals realize their dreams, and that with this tool comes the ability to vitalize and inspire whole civilizations. This is actually true.

   C. Give thanks to the farmer, trucker, storekeeper, nature, the food itself, cookware companies, and anyone else who has made it possible to have these wonderful ingredients and utensils.

   D. A cook can imagine that he or she is composing a symphony or painting a masterpiece as colors, textures, tastes, and smells are arranged into beautiful and dynamic combinations. Anyone who cooks should work to release his or her creativity and intuition. These develop with experience, so be patient and persistent.

   E. Realize that there is always more to learn. One should never become arrogant and think that he or she now knows it all. Be open and learn from everyone. We all have different perspectives and ideas and therefore we all have something to offer.

2. Clean and organize the kitchen and surroundings before, during, and after cooking.

3. Long hair should be tied back to prevent it from catching on fire as well as from falling into the food. Wear a clean apron and roll up long sleeves.

4. Work quickly, calmly, and efficiently, economically making the most of one's time. Avoid munching while cooking as this will really slow things down.

5. Keep other activities and distractions to a minimum and concentrate all energies on the task at hand.

6. When making a menu, first look at all leftovers and older vegetables and use these first. Do not waste any food. Avoid buying more perishables than needed. Check supplies first before going shopping.

7. Develop intuition and common sense in order to appropriately adapt meals to the weather, the season, the people for whom one is cooking, and one's own needs. A cook should be aware of the daily needs and changes of others, his or her own moods, and any other influencing factors for that particular place and time.

8. Keep meals simple. Do not mash together a lot of different ingredients into one dish. Go light on seasonings and use them mainly to draw out and enhance the natural flavors of food.

9. Decorate food beautifully, set the table using appealing tableware, and make the dining area comfortable and aesthetically pleasing. This enhances appetite and the dining experience.

10. Take the time and place to relax, sit down, and peacefully enjoy meals with appreciation. Chew food thoroughly, the saliva helps digestion. Also, it is best not to eat unless one is truly hungry.

8. Grains and Grain Products

Grains:

Grains stored in a cool, dark, dry location, can be kept indefinitely. Use organically grown grains whenever they are available. To retain their maximum energy, leave grains unhusked until just before cooking, if possible.

Before washing grains, spread a handful at a time on a plate, and remove any stones and other debris which may be mixed in. Then, place the grains in a bowl (lightweight stainless-steel mixing bowls are excellent for this), cover with cold water, and very gently stir and rinse off any dirt that floats to the top. Pour out this water, and repeat the above steps until the water remains clear. Then, place the grain in a colander or strainer. Wash quickly to help retain the grain's nutrients.

There are a variety of grains available:

Brown Rice:

Brown rice, being the easiest to digest, is the most suitable grain for daily use. It can be eaten every day, regardless of whether an individual is in the transitional, healing, or standard phase. We eat brown rice at almost every meal. The other grains serve as variations, either as a substitute or as an additional ingredient in a meal. We mainly use four types of rice:

1. *Short-grain:* Short-grain rice is the variety with the hardiest taste and energy, and the most effective one for creating a healthy, balanced condition. Use this one most of the time, especially in the winter.

2. *Medium-grain:* Medium-grain rice is more soft and moist, and is a nice variation.

3. *Long-grain:* Long-grain rice is light and fluffy, excellent for fried rice, and makes a great alternative in the summer and warmer climates.

4. *Sweet rice:* Sweet rice is even more sweet and glutinous than the short grain, and is quite sticky. Sweet rice can be added to other grains periodically for a sweeter taste, and also serves as a base for *ohagi*, mochi, and amazaké.

We recommend pressure-cooking your rice most of the time. This form of preparation cooks the grains more thoroughly, making them easier to digest. Pressure-cooked grains are less soggy, and are sweeter and more healing. Along with the help of a pressure cooker there are two ways to make your grain softer, sweeter, and more digestible:

1. *Non-soaking:* Start cooking the grain very slowly over a low flame, in an uncovered pressure cooker. Do not put any salt in yet so that it will take more time to come to a boil. When it comes to a boil, add the salt, cover, and bring up to pressure (it is up when the gauge hisses). Then, place a heat deflector underneath (make sure the flame is on medium-low) and simmer for 45 to 50 minutes.

2. *Soaking:* Soak the rice (covered with cold water) for 3 to 5 hours or overnight. Place in the pressure cooker (along with the soaking water). This time, add salt and cover right away (otherwise it may turn out too soggy). Put on a medium-high flame and bring up to pressure. When it is up, turn the flame down to medium-low, place a heat deflector underneath, and simmer for 45 to 50 minutes.

Basic Brown Rice (Pressure-Cooked)
(Use every day, the principal food for all conditions.)

3 cups brown rice
3¾–4½ cups spring water
3 pinches sea salt

Pressure-cook following one of the above methods. Let the pressure come down completely before removing the cover. Scoop out the rice, with a wet rice paddle or wooden spoon, into a wooden bowl as you separate and air out the lumps.

The bottom rice can be mixed in if it is not burnt. Keep the brown side turned down and totally covered to help keep it soft. If the bottom is really stuck to the pot, keep a 1-inch layer of rice in the pot, put the lid back on, and let it sit for 20 to 30 minutes. The warmth of the fresh rice will help to loosen and soften the bottom.

Keep the rice covered with a bamboo or sushi mat. This will protect it while letting air circulate. When ready to serve, dish the rice into individual bowls. Serves 6.

Azuki Bean Rice
(Helps strengthen the kidneys and adrenals.)

2½ cups brown rice, washed
½ cup azuki beans, washed
4½ cups spring water
2 pinches sea salt
1 piece kombu, 1½″ long

Boil azuki beans with the kombu in 2 cups of water for 10 to 15 minutes until the water becomes red. Cool the beans until they are lukewarm. Put the rice in the pressure cooker with the beans and their red, boiled juice. Use pressure-cooking method #1 (*Non-soaking*) and follow the directions for *Basic Brown Rice*. Or, soak the rice and beans together overnight and use method #2 (*Soaking*). Serves 6.

Black Soybean Rice

2½ cups brown rice, washed
1½ cup black soybeans
4¼–4½ cups spring water
2 tsps. tamari soy sauce

Place black soybeans on a clean, damp towel. Cover the beans with the towel and rub to remove any dust. (Do not wash or the skins will come off.) Dry-roast beans for several minutes in a skillet, stirring constantly. When the beans begin to split open and the insides are slightly brown, remove and mix with rice in a pressure cooker. Add water and tamari soy sauce. Use *Pressure-cooking Method* #1.

Gomoku Rice

2 cups brown rice
2 Tbsps. diced dried lotus root
2 pieces dried tofu
6 medium diced shiitake mushrooms
2 Tbsps. sliced dried daikon
2 2″-squares diced kombu
1 tsp. finely minced scallion roots
1 large diced carrot
1½ cups spring water per cup of rice
Chopped scallions or parsley for garnish

Dry-roast the rice in a frying pan, stirring gently about 10 to 15 minutes over a low heat. Soak the dried lotus root in warm water for 30 minutes. Soak the dried tofu for 10 min tes, the shiitake for 10 minutes, and the daikon and kombu for 5 minutes each. Dice these ingredients, but do not mince, to obtain ⅓ cup each of the lotus root, tofu, mushrooms, daikon, and kombu. Place roasted rice in a pressure cooker. Add all the other ingredients and mix well. Add a pinch of sea salt per cup of rice. Pressure-cook for 45 to 50 minutes as for regular rice. Then remove the pot from the burner and let it sit 5 minutes or more. Reduce pressure and remove the cover. Garnish with scallions or parsley.

Lotus Seed Rice

(The addition of lotus seeds makes this dish especially strengthening for the lungs and the kidneys.)

2½ cups rice
½ cup lotus seeds
4½ cups spring water
3 pinches sea salt

Wash and soak lotus seeds and rice 3 to 4 hours or overnight. Pressure-cook using method #2 and following the directions for *Basic Brown Rice* (*Pressure-cooked*). Serves 6.

Shiso Rice

2½ cups brown rice, washed
3¾–4½ cups spring water
2 pinches sea salt
¼ cup finely minced shiso leaves

Pressure-cook as for method #1 or #2. When rice is done, remove and place in a wooden bowl. Mix in shiso thoroughly with rice.

Sweet Rice and Chestnuts

2½ cups sweet brown rice, washed
½ cup dried chestnuts
3¾–4½ cups spring water
2–3 pinches sea salt

Wash dried chestnuts after sorting out any discolored ones. Dry-roast in a skillet, on a low flame, for several minutes, stirring constantly. Combine rice and dried, roasted chestnuts in a pressure-cooker. Add water and cook as for *Pressure-cooking Method* #1 or #2.

Sweet Rice and Millet

(Strengthens spleen, pancreas and stomach.)

2 cups sweet rice
1 cup millet

4 cups spring water
3 pinches sea salt

Wash and combine all the ingredients and cook as in *Basic Brown Rice* (*Pressure-cooked*), method #2 (minus the *soaking*) for 40 to 45 minutes. Serves 6.

Other variations include:

1) **2½ cups rice + ½ cup barley (4½ cups water)**
2) **2 cups rice + 1 cup millet (4½ cups water)**
3) **2 cups rice + 1 cup sweet rice**
4) **2½ cups rice + ½ cup wheat berries (soaked overnight)**
5) **2½ cups rice + ½ cup roasted sunflower seeds**
6) **2½ cups rice + ½ cup chick-peas (soaked overnight)**
7) **2 cups rice + 1 cup dried chestnuts**
8) **2 cups rice + 1 cup fresh corn kernels (3 cups water)**
9) **2½ cups rice + ½ cup wild rice**
10) **2½ cups rice + ½ cup roasted walnuts**
11) **2 cups rice + 1 umeboshi plum (instead of salt)**
12) **Bancha tea instead of water**
13) **2½ cups rice + 1 cup squash**
14) **2½ cups rice + ½ cup roasted black or yellow soybeans**

You can also boil the rice once in a while. Boiling does not give the strength of pressure-cooking but it is a great alternative when you want something lighter, more yin, and to add some variety. When eating boiled rice, make sure to chew well. You can dry-roast the rice before boiling it for variation.

Basic Brown Rice (Boiled)

2 cups brown rice, washed
4 cups spring water
2 pinches sea salt

Put washed rice into a pot (preferably with a heavy lid) with water and salt. Bring to a boil, then lower the flame, place a heat deflector underneath, and simmer for about 1 hour or until all the water has been absorbed. Wet a wooden spoon or rice paddle and dish out the rice into a wooden bowl. Cover with a sushi or bamboo mat. Serves 4.

Option: Roast the rice in a skillet till golden brown before boiling it. This gives more flavor. Gently stir the grains with a wooden spoon to prevent burning.

When a person is not feeling well, soft rice is often recommended. It is more soothing and is easier on the digestive system. Soft rice can be accompanied by an umeboshi plum in cases of poor digestion. Even for people in good health, this makes a delicious porridge. Omit the salt to make a perfect food for babies and young children.

Soft Rice (Plain)

1 cup brown rice
5 cups water
1 pinch sea salt

Cook as in *Basic Brown Rice* (*Pressure-cooked*). Soft rice can also be prepared by simmering it overnight over a low flame and a heat deflector. In this case, use 10 cups of water to every cup of rice. Serves 5.

The following dish of soft rice with miso may be eaten often, particularly in the winter, or by persons suffering from weak digestion.

Ojiya (Soft Rice with Miso)

2 cups leftover cooked brown rice
4–5 cups spring water
2 level tsps. miso
1 strip kombu, 1½" long, washed, soaked, and sliced
3–4 sliced scallions

Place the kombu on the bottom of a pot or pressure cooker. Add the rice and water and bring them to a boil or up to pressure. Turn the flame to low, place a deflector underneath, and simmer or pressure-cook for ½ hour. Add 1 tablespoon or so of water to the miso and stir it in until the miso becomes a purée. Uncover the rice (wait until the pressure is down if using a pressure cooker), and then put it back onto the stove. Mix in the miso, simmer for another 3 to 5 minutes, then turn off the flame. Garnish with sliced scallions and serve immediately. Serves 4 to 5.

Rice Cream with Nori and Umeboshi
(Rice cream is a dish with special healing qualities. It helps purify blood and lymph.)

1 cup dry-roasted brown rice
3–6 cups spring water
1 pinch sea salt
1 sheet toasted nori
1 umeboshi plum
Cheesecloth

Pressure-cook with salt and water for 1 hour following directions for *Basic Brown Rice* (*Pressure-cooked*). Make a sack out of clean cheesecloth. Cool off the cooked rice, place some inside the sack and squeeze out as much of the creamy liquid as you can. Reheat and serve with nori and an umeboshi plum. The leftover pulp can be eaten separately or added to soup or vegetable dishes.

Especially good condiments for this dish are gomashio, umeboshi, toasted nori, green nori flakes, tekka, and shiso leaves. Serves 2.

Musubi (Rice Ball)
(Great for lunches, picnics, and trips, rice balls are also a very strengthening, stabilizing way to eat rice.)

1 cup cooked short-grain (sticks well) brown rice
2 quarters of a nori sheet (a sheet cut in half then half again)
1 pinch sea salt
1 umeboshi plum (or ½ if it is large)

Toast nori by passing it over an open flame a few times, until it becomes green but not so much that it becomes crisp and crinkly. Tear it into 4 pieces.

Wet hands (to prevent the rice from sticking to them) in a bowl of salted water. While holding the rice, stick an umeboshi plum in the middle (the pit may be removed if desired). Tightly mold the rice around the plum in an English-muffin shape or a flat triangle and put it on a plate.

Fig. 11 Rice Balls

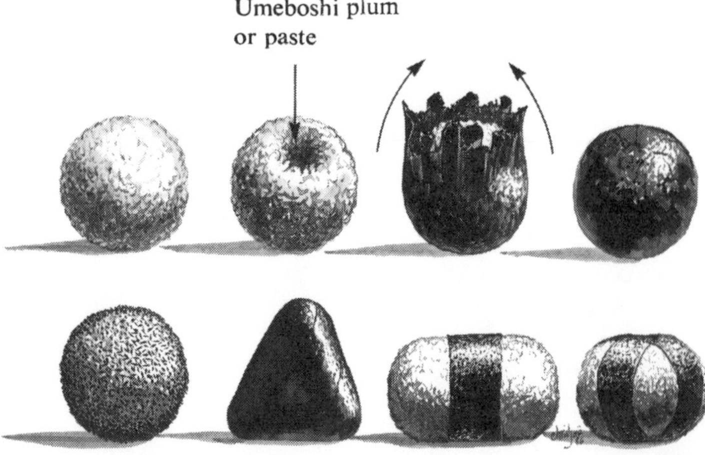

With dry hands, use a quarter sheet of nori (the shiny side on the outside), to cover each side of the rice ball. Firmly mold it on. The rice ball is now ready to eat, or pack it up and take it on a trip to consume later. Serves 1.

Frying is a delicious way to prepare leftover rice. This method may be used once or twice a week while on a healing diet. If oil must be avoided, sauté the vegetables in a small amount of simmering water instead. All types of vegetables may be used, but in cases of reproductive disorders, hard leafy greens and sweet vegetables such as carrots, onions, and cabbage should be emphasized. Below are two recipes.

Basic Fried Rice

4 cups cooked short-grain brown rice
Kernels from 4 ears of corn, cooked
1 onion, sliced in thin half-moons
1 Tbsp. dark (toasted) sesame oil or a small amount of spring water
Tamari soy sauce

Sauté the onion in a skillet a few minutes, being careful not to let it burn. Add rice, layering it over the onion. Cover the skillet, and cook approximately 15 minutes, adding a little water to prevent burning. Add the corn and a sprinkling of tamari soy sauce, mix well, and cook 5 to 10 minutes more. Garnish with chopped scallions or parsley. Serves 3 to 4.

Summer Fried Rice

3 cups cooked brown rice
1/4 cup celery, cut on thin diagonal
1/2 cup carrot, matchsticks
1/2 cup fresh sweet corn
2 Tbsps. minced parsley, garnish
1 Tbsps. dark sesame oil
Optional: Tamari soy sauce

Heat oil in a skillet. Sauté celery 1 minute. Add corn and carrots. Place cooked rice on top of vegetables. Cover, reduce flame to low, and cook 7 to 10 minutes, or until vegetables and rice are hot.

Season lightly with tamari soy sauce, and cook 3 to 4 minutes more. Add parsley, mix well, and cook 1 to 2 minutes more. Place in serving bowl. (If rice is dry, you may add several drops of spring water at beginning of cooking to moisten.)

Norimaki (Sushi)
(Sushi rolls are handy as appetizers, snacks, and for traveling, and have a very decorative appearance.)

1½ cups cooked short-grain (sticks best) brown rice
1 sheet nori
1 carrot, cut into several lengthwise strips
2–3 uncut (except for the roots) scallions
1″ boiling water in a pot
¼–½ tsp. umeboshi paste
1 pinch sea salt

Add a pinch of salt (for brighter vegetable colors) to the boiling water and cook the carrot strips until they are soft. Remove the strips and let them drain. Next, boil the scallions (cut off the roots) for just a second, but not until they loose the bright green color, then remove and drain them.

Meanwhile, toast a sheet of nori by passing it over an open flame (on the dull side only for easier rolling) until it is green but not so much that it is overly crisp and crinkly.

Place a sushi mat on a cutting board, and lay the sheet of nori on top of it. The halfway fold of the nori should be horizontal to the cook. With wet hands, evenly press a ¼-inch layer of rice onto the nori, leaving ½ to ¾ inch of the top edge (the side away from one) and ¼ inch of the bottom edge uncovered. Then, make a horizontal indentation in the rice 1 inch up from the bottom of the nori and spread the umeboshi paste inside the length of it. Then press 1 to 3 carrot strips and the scallions (again horizontally) on top of the paste.

Next, slowly roll the mat and its contents upwards, pressing firmly upon the rice and other ingredients. Try to tuck the vegetables underneath while rolling. Wet the top edge of the uncovered nori (to help in sealing) and complete the roll.

With dry hands, place the roll with the sealed edge underneath, wet a vegetable knife (to prevent the rice from sticking to it for smooth, easy cutting), and slowly, carefully and firmly cut the roll into 1-inch slices. Place the slices onto a plate with the inside turned upward to show their beautiful design, then decorate, and serve. Makes 5 pieces.

Mochi is a traditional Japanese dish which is eaten on festive occasions. Mochi cakes or squares are made of pounded sweet rice. Several pieces in miso soup can help strengthen the intestines.

Mochi (Homemade)

4 cups sweet rice
4 cups water
4 pinches sea salt
A handful of sweet rice flour (optional)

Cook as in *Basic Brown Rice* (*Pressure-cooked*). When done, in a wooden bowl, vigorously pound the rice with a large wooden pestle (which is moistened initially and from time to time to prevent the rice from sticking to it) until all the grains are crushed and form a smooth, sticky mass. This may take a half hour. Sprinkle some flour onto a baking sheet and layer the rice on top (up to 1-inch thick). Dry this for 1 to 2 days and then store it in the refrigerator.

To serve, cut the mochi into small pieces and toast them in a skillet with or without oil until they become soft. This only takes a few minutes. (Turn them over when they are half done so that both sides toast evenly.) Serve them with some raw grated daikon with a few drops of tamari soy sauce added. The daikon helps in digestion of the mochi. Serves 5 to 6.

Fortunately, mochi can now be purchased in some natural food stores. In this case, all that is needed is to toast it for a few minutes in the oven or in a dry frying pan over a medium-low flame to avoid burning.

Ohagi

Ohagi are balls or cakes of slightly pounded sweet rice which are coated with tamari soy sauce, roasted and ground nuts or seeds, purėed sweet azuki beans, or purėed, cooked dried chestnuts. Makes a delicious snack, party, or meal-time dish.

To prepare, cook sweet rice in the same way as for mochi. When done, pound the cooked rice with a wooden pestle only until the grain is half-crushed. This may take 15 to 20 minutes. Form this "dough" into small balls or flat cakes and roll in various coatings.

Millet:

Millet is a more yang grain, being small, round, and more alkaline. It is good for the spleen and pancreas, it helps to settle an acidic stomach, and it gives warmth. For helping to relieve blood glucose disorders millet can be considered as a major grain after rice.

Millet cooks fairly quickly and comes out very soft, so it can, but does not need to be pressure-cooked. It can also be cooked in combination with rice, using 10 to 15 percent millet. Millet can be made either light and fluffy, or moist and creamy like a porridge. The fluffy style can be a little dry, so it can often be eaten with a sauce or cooked with other ingredients. A standard combination uses squash. Other common companions are vegetables like carrots and onions as well as roasted seeds.

Millet Porridge

1 cup millet, washed
4 cups boiling water
1 pinch sea salt

Bring salt and water to a boil. Carefully pour the millet into the pot of boiling water. Bring to a boil again, turn the flame to low, place a heat deflector underneath, cover, and simmer for 30 minutes. Serves 3.

Millet and Squash

2 cups millet
1 small winter squash
2½ cups spring water
2 pinches sea salt

Wash millet and dry-roast in a skillet approximately 5 to 8 minutes, or until lightly browned. Place the millet and squash

Millet and Vegetables

2 cups millet, washed and dry-roasted
Kernels from 2–3 ears fresh sweet corn
½ cup diced carrots
¼ cup diced burdock
¼ cup diced celery
¼ cup diced onions
½ cup diced cooked seitan
3 cups spring water
Chopped parsley for garnish

Put the millet and vegetables in a pot and add water. Salt is not necessary as there is tamari soy sauce in the seitan. Cover the pot and place over medium heat. When simmering, place a flame deflector under the pot. Cook approximately 30 minutes. Place all ingredients in a serving bowl and garnish with chopped parsley and serve. Serves 4.

Barley:

Barley is usually used in combination with other grains (such as rice) and vegetables. It is very mild tasting and lends itself easily to this. Cook it just like rice. It is light and has a cooling, calming energy.

Barley Porridge

1 cup barley (soak 6–8 hours)
4–5 cups spring water
1 pinch sea salt
Several parsley sprigs, or chopped scallions

Boil as in *Basic Brown Rice* (*Boiled*). Simmer for 1¼ to 1½ hours or until soft. Garnish with the parsley or scallions. Serves 5.

Brown Rice and Hato Mugi

2½ cups brown rice, washed
½ cup hato mugi, washed
3¾–4½ cups spring water
3 pinches sea salt

Cook as for *Pressure-cooking Method* #1 or #2.

Buckwheat:

Buckwheat can grow in a very cold climate and has a short growing season. This grain gives strength, generates heat, and is good for the lungs, kidneys and bladder. It is a great winter food.

Buckwheat can be cooked just like millet as it also cooks quickly and is a very soft grain. Below is a recipe for creamy kasha (buckwheat).

Creamy Kasha

1 cup buckwheat groats
2 scallions
5 cups spring water
1 pinch sea salt

Wash the buckwheat and put it into a pot. Add cold water and sea salt and bring to a boil. Then turn the flame down to low, place a flame deflector underneath and cook for 20 to 30 minutes. Wash and slice the scallions for a garnish. Serves 3.

Buckwheat Salad

1 cup buckwheat groats
½ cup chopped, drained sauerkraut (save liquid)
1 cup steamed, chopped kale

2 Tbsps. finely chopped parsley
2 cups spring water plus the sauerkraut juice
Pinch sea salt

Wash the buckwheat and dry-roast it for several minutes in a frying pan. Bring the water and the drained sauerkraut juice to a boil. Add the buckwheat and salt to the boiling liquid. Cover and cook for 20 minutes.

Sauté finely chopped parsley in a very small amount of water. Mix the parsley with the buckwheat. Mix in the steamed, chopped kale and chopped sauerkraut. Serve with a dressing made of 1 teaspoon tamari soy sauce and 1 teaspoon squeezed ginger juice. Serves 3.

Dressing

1/8–1/4 cup tamari soy sauce
1 tsp. fresh-squeezed ginger juice
1 cup cooking water from tempeh

Mix together and serve over salad.

Oats:

Oats have more protein and fat than other grains. Therefore, while they are helpful to produce more warmth in the body, they should not be taken on a daily basis as they can cause a buildup of mucus. Use about two times a week maximum during the initial healing stage, and use whole oats whenever possible.

Whole Oats

1 cup whole oats
5 cups spring water
1 pinch sea salt
1 strip kombu, 3″–6″

Wash and soak oats for 3 hours or overnight. Add kombu (it helps to cut the fat in the oats) and pressure-cook 2 hours, or boil just like brown rice. If boiling, slowly simmer over a low flame for three or more hours or overnight. Small cubes of winter squash can also be cooked along with the oats for a sweet flavor. Serves 3.

Scotch Oats

1 cup Scotch oats
3 cups water

1 pinch sea salt
1 strip kombu, 2″–4″

Combine water, salt, and kombu, and bring to a boil. Wash and dry-roast oats in a skillet for 5 minutes, stirring with a wooden spoon over a medium-low flame. Then, carefully pour oats into the boiling water. Bring back to a boil, turn heat to medium-low, place a flame deflector underneath, and cook for about 30 to 40 minutes. Serves 2.

Oatmeal (Rolled Oats)

1 cup rolled oats
3 cups water
1 pinch sea salt
Optional: 1 strip kombu, 2″–4″, kombu, soaked 20 minutes

If using kombu, cut it into ½-inch pieces. Bring water to a boil, including kombu soaking water. Add salt and oats. (They can be toasted or not.) Reduce heat to medium-low, place a flame deflector underneath, and simmer for 20 minutes or more.

Wheat:

Wheat berries are harder to digest than other grains. They should always be soaked beforehand. Make sure you chew really well in order to insure good digestion.

Pressure-cook like rice except that the wheat berries need to be soaked for several hours or overnight. You may also need to cook them an extra 10 to 15 minutes. Use twice as much water as grain.

Wheat also comes in the form of bulgur, which has been partially boiled, dried, and then ground; and couscous, which has been refined and cracked. Both of these wheat products are convenient, as they cook very quickly, especially couscous. However, they should not be used as staple foods since a great deal of nutrition is lost in their processing. Use them as an occasional treat and for variety.

Azuki Beans with Wheat Berries

(See chapter on *Beans* for recipe.)

Brown Rice with Wheat Berries

2½ cups brown rice, washed
½ cup wheat berries, soaked 4–6 hours
3¾–4½ cups spring water
3 pinches sea salt

Cook as for *Pressure-cooking Method* **#1**.

Bulgur and Vegetables

1 cup bulgur
¼ cup each diced onions, carrots, and celery
2–2¼ cups spring water
1 pinch sea salt

Bring salt and water to a boil. Meanwhile, wash and dice the vegetables and layer them (onions on the bottom, then celery, and finally carrots on top) in another pot. Add some water (just enough to cover the vegetables) and simmer until they are soft. Then, add the bulgur, pour the boiling water on top, cover, and bring to a boil again. Turn the flame to low and simmer for 20 minutes. Serves 3.

Boiled Couscous

1 cup couscous
2½ cups spring water
1 pinch sea salt
Optional: **1 tsp. sesame oil**

Bring the water, salt, and optional oil to a boil. Pour in the couscous, turn the flame to low, cover, and simmer for 5 minutes. Add some garnish or sauce. Serves 2.

Corn:

The corn eaten by the native American Indians was much hardier, stronger, smaller, and nutritious than most of the commercial corn available today. This grain was more effective in maintaining one's health, particularly strengthening the heart and blood vessels.

During the healing stage use only corn dishes that have been cooked whole at the beginning, such as whole corn dishes and traditional *masa*, *tortillas*, and so on. Avoid dishes that have been ground previous to any cooking, as they may cause a buildup of mucus.

There are five main types of corn available today:

1. *Sweet corn*—The regular corn on the cob.
2. *Dent corn*—Corn with dented kernels used for making cornmeal.
3. *Flour corn*—Starchy variety used in Latin American cooking.
4. *Flint corn*—Starchy variety used in Latin America Cooking.
5. *Popcorn.*

Corn on the Cob (Boiled)

Desired number of ears of fresh corn
A large pot of water
Umeboshi paste

Trim away the dry, outer leaves of the corn, but keep the fresher inner wrapping intact. Chop off the excess straggly husk ends and silk hairs on the top end of the corn. Put sea salt in the water and bring the pot to a boil. Drop the corn in and boil for about 10 minutes. Take out the corn and serve. After unhusking individual ears of corn, umeboshi paste can be rubbed on it if desired. Strain out any leftover silk hairs in the liquid with an oil skimmer and use this liquid for soup stock.

Corn Grits

1 cup corn grits, washed
3 cups spring water
1 pinch sea salt

Bring water and salt to a boil. Slowly add corn grits, stirring constantly to avoid lumping. Cover, reduce flame to low, and simmer 20 to 30 minutes. Garnish and serve.

Dried Whole Corn (Dent)

2 cups whole, dried dent corn
8 cups spring water
2 pinches sea salt
1 cup sifted wood ash

Wash and soak the corn overnight. Put the corn, 4 cups of water, and the wood ash (no salt) in a pressure cooker. Cook for 30 to 45 minutes. When the corn is done, put it into a colander or strainer. Rinse out all the ash and remove the corn skins. (If the skins are not loose enough, cook again with more ashes for another 10 minutes.) Pressure-cook the un-hulled corn for 1 hour in a clean pot with salt and 4 more cups of water. The corn can be served as it is, or used as a base for other corn recipes (see below). Serves 4 to 6.

Masa (Corn Dough)

4 cups whole, dried flint corn
8–10 cups water initially and 8 more cups later
1 cup sifted wood ash
3–4 pinches sea salt

Follow the directions in *Dried Whole Corn* but use 8 to 10 cups of water in the beginning and 8 more cups after the corn is hulled. Take out and cool the corn. Grind it in a hand grinder (not a blender). Knead this for about 15 minutes. Moisten it with a little water if it is too dry. If not using the dough immediately, store it in the refrigerator (up to a week). This is the base for many corn recipes such as arepas, tortillas, cereals, and so on.

Arepas

3 cups masa corn dough (see above recipe)
Boiling water
Water to help shape the dough
2–3 pinches sea salt
1 Tbsp. sesame oil
Optional: ½ cup roasted sesame seeds

Knead the dough while mixing in salt and optional sesame seeds. It should feel like bread dough. If it is too dry, add a little water, and if too wet, add more dough or let it sit and dry for a few minutes. Separate it into balls which are molded into English-muffin shapes, except a little flatter. Boil some water, put the balls in, and remove them when they rise to the top.

Heat some oil in a skillet, place the arepas inside, cover, and cook them over a low flame for about 15 to 20 minutes. (Turn them over halfway through to cook the other side.) If desired, this is the time to slit them open and stuff them with beans and/or vegetables. Serves 4 to 6.

Grain Products:

During the initial healing period it is better to avoid flour or refined-grain products altogether. This is particularly so for any dry, roasted, or baked items such as bread, crackers, granola, and others. However, boiled, whole-grain flour products may be used occasionally for variety, including noodles, fu, and seitan.

1. Noodles are a great snack and cook up very quickly. There are several types which are now available in most natural food stores.

   A. *Soba*—Long, thin, Oriental buckwheat noodles.
      1) Buckwheat with/without wheat in varying amounts
      2) Jinenjo soba (contains jinenjo flour)

3) *Ito* soba—extra thin and light
4) *Ramen*—Instant noodles

B. *Udon*—Long, Oriental whole wheat noodles.

1) Thicker than soba and contains whole wheat and sometimes unbleached, sifted white flour
2) *Somen*—Very thin wheat noodles
3) Ramen—Instant noodles

C. *Pasta*—Wheat alone or in combination with other grain flours.

1) Spaghetti
2) Shells
3) Spirals
4) Elbows
5) Ribbons
6) Ziti
7) Rigatoni
8) Linguini
9) Lasagna
10) Alphabets, etc.

Buy these noodles, especially the ramen and pasta, from natural food stores. The ramen bought in Oriental shops may contain animal fats, sugar, MSG, chemicals, additives, and food coloring. Pasta bought in a regular store usually contain eggs which are best avoided.

To cook noodles, place them in a large pot of boiling water. (Too little water causes them to clump together.) As the pasta is added, stir and separate the noodles with a long chopstick to prevent them from lying side by side in a parallel fashion, otherwise they will stick together. (This precaution is basically for long thin noodles such as udon and soba.)

Keep the flame high and add a little cold water each time the pot comes to a boil, until the noodles are soft (usually about 3 times). Or, turn the flame down a bit after adding the noodles, and simmer until they are cooked. The first method is preferred as the noodles come out more firm and crisp. When done, the inside is the same color as the outside. Drain them in a colander and immediately run cold water over them. This helps to keep them from clumping together.

Avoid making noodles too soggy, especially if they are later going to be reheated or fried. Pay special attention to the somen and Ito soba, as they cook up very quickly and are absolutely horrible when soft and mushy.

Add a pinch of salt when boiling pasta. (Udon and soba already contain salt so they don't need it.) The leftover noodle water can be used in soup stocks.

Noodles in Broth

1 pack udon or soba noodles previously boiled
1 1″ to 2″ piece kombu
1 shiitake mushroom, soaked and sliced
4 cups spring water, including shiitake soaking water
½ cake tofu, cut into small cubes
3 Tbsps. tamari soy sauce
1–2 sheets toasted nori, cut into small pieces
3 chopped scallions

Make a soup stock by bringing kombu, shiitake, and water to a boil, and simmering for 5 minutes. Take out the kombu and shiitake. Boil the tofu cubes and take them out when they rise to the top. Add the tamari and simmer for 5 to 7 minutes. Put in some noodles (only add what you are immediately going to eat and keep the rest aside) until they become warm, then dish them out into individual bowls. Place some tofu, shiitake slices, nori, and scallions on top of each bowl, pour some broth over them and serve.

For variation:

1) Add different kinds of sea vegetables, root, or green vegetables into the broth, boil them until soft, and add the tamari soy sauce.
2) Add different kinds of sea vegetables, and/or boiled, sautéed, or thinly sliced raw vegetables as a garnish. Roasted seeds, fu (soak and boil it in the broth previously, as was done with the tofu above), cooked seitan and tempeh, and grated daikon or ginger can also be added.
3) As a general rule, anything can be added as long as there is a sea vegetable in the broth, and a pungent item in the garnish. This would include scallions, diced cooked onions, chives, or daikon, as they help digestion.

Zaru Soba

Soba, previously boiled
1 Tbsp. tamari soy sauce
1 Tbsp. brown rice vinegar
4 Tbsps. kombu soup stock

Chopped scallions
Nori, toasted and cut into thin strips

Place soba noodles onto an individual serving plate and place a few strips of nori on top. (In Japan they have special individual bamboo serving "plates" which allows soba to drain.) Combine tamari soy sauce, rice vinegar, kombu stock, and scallions into a small bowl to make a dip for the noodles. Make a dip for each person.

Fried Noodles (Water-Sautéed)

4 cups spring water
1 package soba or udon noodles
2 cups shredded cabbage
1–2 Tbsps. tamari soy sauce
½ cup sliced scallions

Boil the noodles, rinse them under cold water, and drain. Place a small amount of spring water in a frying pan and add the cabbage. Put the cooked noodles on top of the cabbage, cover the pan, and cook over low heat for 5 to 7 minutes, or until the noodles are warm. Add the tamari soy sauce and mix the noodles and vegetables well. Do not stir the ingredients together until this time; they should be left to cook peacefully until the very end. Cook for several minutes longer and add the scallions at the very end. Serve hot or cold.

2. Seitan is a protein-rich wheat product. It is made from the gluten of hard spring or winter wheat flours.

Seitan
(Seitan can also be bought in natural food stores. Avoid ones that have been heavily spiced if in the process of healing.)

3½ lbs. whole wheat flour (spring or winter)
8–9 cups of water

Place the flour into a large stainless-steel mixing bowl, and gradually add the water. Form a dough and knead it for 5 to 15 minutes until it becomes stiff and earlobe consistency.

Submerge the dough in water and let it sit for 5 to 10 minutes. Then knead and separate the dough in the water until the liquid is full of bran and starch.

Drain the seitan in a colander which is placed inside a large pot. (If desired, save the soaking water, starch, and bran. It can be used to thicken soups, sauces, stews, puddings, and so on, as well as for pancakes, waffles, and sourdough starter.) Add cold water to the pot and start to knead all the bran out of the gluten.

If this water also becomes overly branny, add fresh water. (Save this bran water as well, if desired.) Start to take small pieces of the gluten, one at a time, and wash the bran out of them. They can be rinsed under the tap. (Some remaining flecks of bran here and there is all right. It need not be prefectly bran-free.)

When finished, separate the gluten into several pieces and drop them into a pot of boiling water until they rise to the surface. (Or, deep-fry them until they puff up and turn golden brown. Try it this way when no longer healing; it is delicous.)

Cook the seitan further if desired. Put a piece of kombu, seitan, ⅓ to ½ cup tamari soy sauce, and 6 cups of spring water into a pot, bring it to a boil, turn flame to low, cover, and simmer for about a half hour. Eat as is or add to other dishes, including soups, salads, vegetables, stews, grains, and the like.

Seitan Stew

2 cups cooked seitan, sliced
1 strip kombu, soaked and sliced
1 cup onions, cut into ¼-inch-thick half-moons
½ cup celery, cut into ¼-inch-thick diagonals
1 cup carrots, cut in chunks
1 to 1½ cups cooked seitan, cut into chunks
3 to 4 cups kombu-tamari water from cooking seitan
½ 1½ cups starch-bran water from cooking seitan, or 1 rounded Tbsp. kuzu, dissolved in 1 cup water
Chopped scallions or parsley for garnish

Put the kombu in a pot. Add the onions, celery, carrots, and seitan. Pour in the kombu-tamari cooking water and bring to a boil. Cover and lower the heat. Simmer until all the vegetables are soft, about 30 to 40 minutes. Add the starch-bran water or kuzu to thicken, and stir well. Let simmer for another 15 to 20 minutes. Garnish with chopped scallions or parsley and serve.

Seitan, Onions, Corn and Sauerkraut

3 cups cooked seitan, sliced
1 large Spanish onion, sliced into ¼-inch-thick rings
½ cup sauerkraut, chopped

1 cup fresh sweet corn
1 cup seitan-tamari cooking water
2 tsps. chopped parsley

Layer in a skillet, onions, corn, seitan, and sauerkraut in that order. Add seitan-tamari water. Cover and bring to a boil. Reduce flame to medium-low and simmer 15 to 20 minutes or so, until the onions are soft and tender. Garnish with chopped parsley.

3. Fu is also a by-product of wheat gluten. It looks like a cracker and is packaged and available in natural food stores. Fu comes in flat sheets or thick rounds which are available in small or large sizes.

Fu and Vegetables

1 pkg. fu, soaked and sliced
1 cup broccoli spears
½ cup onion, chunks
¼ cup carrot, matchsticks
¼ cup cabbage, chunks
Water
Tamari soy sauce

Place fu, onions, carrots, and cabbage in a pot. Half-cover with water. Bring to a boil. Reduce the flame to medium-low, cover, and simmer several minutes, until the vegetables are almost done. Add broccoli and simmer 2 to 3 minutes more. Mildly season with tamari soy sauce and simmer until broccoli is tender but still bright green.

Fig. 12 Fu

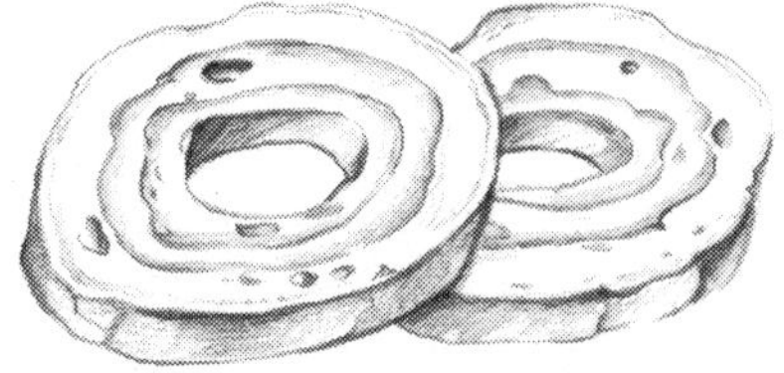

4. Sourdough bread. When healing, it is best to abstain from baked flour products, as mentioned before, but if you do crave some, natural, unyeasted sourdough bread is best.

Yeast is not recommended as it can cause indigestion, and can weaken the intestines.

Hard spring or winter wheat flours make the best bread as they contain much gluten which helps the bread rise. Any other flour can be added in smaller proportions for a variation in taste, as can any cooked grains. (Cooked grains that have already gone sour can replace the sourdough starter.)

Before making a sourdough bread, you first need to make a starter.

Sourdough Starter

1 cup whole wheat flour
1–1½ cups well or spring water

Put flour and water into a bowl and mix them into a thick batter or porridge-like consistency, adding more flour or water as needed. Cover with a damp towel, and let it sit for 2 to 4 days at room temperature. When it bubbles and becomes sour, it is ready to use.

Sourdough Bread (2 Loaves)

5 cups whole wheat flour
1 cup sourdough starter (or sour seitan water)
2 cups water
1 tsp. sea salt

Mix the starter, water, and 2½ cups of the flour. Let the mixture sit uncovered in a warm place for an hour or so until it rises.

(At this point, half of this batter can be saved for an ongoing starter which can be used continually by adding to and recycling it every week; the longer it has been around the better the bread. If not baking one week, mix in a few spoonfuls of flour and water just to keep the starter going and to prevent it from spoiling. This should be stored in the refrigerator.)

Add the salt and remaining flour, form into a dough, and on a floured board, start kneading the bread, about 350 to 400 times. The more it is kneaded the better it will rise, as the bread gets more and more elastic, glutenous, and smooth. This is the secret to non-yeasted breads.

Place dough into a lightly oiled bowl, cover with a damp towel, and let it sit overnight at room temperature.

The next morning, punch the dough down, knead it for a few minutes, and divide it in half. Place the halves into two oiled bread pans, and with a knife, make a lengthwise slit down the center of the tops. The slit helps to give the bread some room to grow and lets steam escape. Place the pans in a very warm place and let them sit for another 2 to 3 hours or until the bread rises and the slits begin to open.

Make the slits deeper and take an oiled rubber spatula and pull the bread away from the sides of the pans. Bake at 350° to 375° F. for about an hour, or until the bread forms a beautiful brown crust.

Insert a chopstick or fork into the bread and pull it out again. If no flour sticks to it, the bread is done. Also, when tapping the bottom, a hollow sound will be heard if the bread is finished. Remove from the pans and let the loaves cool on a bread rack for several hours. Eating the bread while it is still hot may cause an upset stomach. Keep loaves in a cool, dark place, wrapped in a clean cotton cloth or towel.

Slice with a bread knife. If the bread becomes hard, simply steam the number of slices desired for a few minutes. They will become moist and appear freshly baked.

Steamed Bread

Slice bread and place it in a steamer basket. Steam several minutes until soft and hot, but not so long that it becomes soggy. After the water comes to a boil, reduce the flame so that the water simmers gently. This will prevent the water from bubbling up and soaking the bread.

9. Soups

Soup at the beginning of a meal prepares the digestive system for all the following dishes. Just about anything can be put into a soup. Practically all types of grains, beans and their products, vegetables, sea vegetables, and occasionally, fish, can be used.

Soups can be adapted seasonally (and be either warming or cooling), and can add contrast to the rest of the meal. There are some general guidelines on deciding what kind of soup to use.

In the winter, make more hearty stews and thick soups with more root vegetables, grains, or beans, and use more salt. In the summer, make lighter soups with less ingredients and more liquid, more greens, tofu, and so on. Also make greater use of clear or light tamari-broth soups in hot weather.

For all types of arthritis, miso soup with a variety of vegetables, particularly daikon and green leafy vegetables, should be eaten on a daily basis.

Sweet vegetables such as carrots, onions, squash, parsnips, and cabbage can be used individually or together to make delicious sweet-tasting soups.

Care should be taken to balance soup with the rest of the meal. Some examples are:

1. Make a bean soup for a light meal lacking in more protein-rich dishes such as beans, tempeh, or natto.

2. Make a sweet-vegetable soup (squash, carrots, parsnips, etc.) if the meal is lacking this sweet taste.

3. Make a root-vegetable soup if the meal is mostly greens and vice versa.

4. Make a grain soup to balance a more light meal.

5. Use finely chopped vegetables if the meal contains all big chunks and vice versa.

6. Use a color in the soup which is not represented in the meal.

7. If not making miso soup, miso can be added somewhere else in the meal.

Use a ladle to serve soups. This can be kept on a plate on the counter next to the soup pot or in a bowl during the course of the meal, ready to be used whenever needed.

Especially during the first few months, it is recommended that every day one meal should contain miso soup (unless soft miso rice is eaten that day). Also, every day, at least one soup should contain sea vegetables. Garnishes are important (parsley or scallions) to balance soups as well as for decoration.

1. *Miso soup:* Miso is an indispensible part of the macrobiotic diet. It gives vitality, strengthens the digestive system and blood quality, and improves assimilation of carbohydrates. When healing, eat a small amount every day, particularly in miso soup.

   Miso is salty so care must be taken to avoid consuming too much of it at one time. To use, add a flat teaspoonful per cup of liquid, dissolving the miso in a small amount of liquid before adding it to the soup.

   Miso should be added at the end of cooking, after all the ingredients have softened, and generally should not be boiled as otherwise many valuable healing enzymes are destroyed. However, it is important that the soup be simmered for a few minutes after the miso is added to help the body assimilate it. If this is not done, tightness can arise.

   The recipes below are primarily for mugi (barley) miso, but Hatcho (all soybean) miso may be used on occasion, especially in the winter.

Basic Miso Soup

Wakame or kombu, soaked and sliced
½ cup onions, cut in crescents
½ cup carrots, sliced in half-moons
4 cups spring water
4 level tsps. miso
Scallion or parsley garnish

Soak wakame or kombu for 10 minutes and slice. Boil the slices in water, cutting vegetables in the meantime. Add the vegetables to the boiling water and cook until they are soft, about 10 minutes. Dilute and purée the miso with some of the soup water, turn down the flame, and when the soup has stopped bubbling, gently add and stir the miso purée into the soup. Simmer for 3 to 4 minutes and serve with a garnish.
It is important that the soup be light and energetic by keeping

vegetables fresh and crispy, being careful not to overcook them.

Daikon-Shiitake Miso Soup

1 cup daikon, cut any way you want
2–3 shiitake mushrooms, soaked, de-stemmed and sliced
¼–½ cup wakame soaked and sliced
4 cups water
1¼–1½ Tbsps. pureed barley (mugi) miso
Scallions or parsley garnish

Follow the same recipe directions as for *Basic Miso Soup* (add shiitake first and cook 5 minutes or so before adding daikon).

Other miso soup variations:

1) **Onion and Daikon Miso Soup:** 2 onions, ½ cup daikon, and about 4 inches of wakame.
2) **Mustard Green Miso Soup:** 1 onion, 2 to 4 mustard-green leaves, and about 4 inches of wakame or kombu.
3) **Miso Soup with Root Vegetables:** 1 carrot, 1 onion, ¼ rutabaga, 1 stalk celery, and about 3 inches of wakame or kombu.
4) **Miso Soup with Squash and Onions:** 2 onions, 1 cup winter squash, and about 3 inches of wakame or kombu.
5) **Miso Soup with Roots and Greens:** Use either carrots and carrot tops, daikon and daikon leaves, radish and radish tops, or turnip and turnip greens, with wakame or kombu. Onions could also be added, but are optional.
6) **Miso Soup with Shiitake and Greens:** 1 to 3 shiitake mushrooms, 3 to 5 leaves of green leafy vegetable, and 5 inches of wakame or kombu.
7) **Miso Soup with Tofu:** ½ cake tofu, choice of vegetables, wakame or kombu.
8) **Tempeh Miso Soup:** ½ package of tempeh, 2 onions, and 4 inches of wakame.
9) **Miso Soup with Fu:** 3 sheets flat fu and 1 leek in a kombu stock.
10) **Dulse Miso Soup:** Use dulse in place of wakame or kombu. Try dulse with cabbage and carrots.

2. *Clear broth or tamari soy sauce soup:* Light soups are very appealing in the hot summer months or when the rest of the meal

is more heavy. A stronger tamari broth is very good as a standard supper soup for noodles, but care should be taken that the soup does not have a markedly salty taste.

For a clear soup, make a stock and add the vegetables and some form of salt. The following guidelines apply to the making of soup stock:

A. To retain the clear color of the stock, use a pinch of sea salt per cup of liquid.
B. A darker soup can be made by using 2 to 3 tablespoons of tamari soy sauce for every four cups of liquid.
C. For occasional use, 1 flat tablespoon of umeboshi paste or 2 umeboshi plums for 4 cups of liquid will give an attractive pink coloring to a soup.

Clear Broth Soup

1 cake tofu, cubed
1 bunch watercress, washed, par-boiled ½ minute
½ cup carrot, cut in thin rounds
4 cups kombu-shiitake soup stock
2–3 Tbsps. tamari soy sauce

Bring soup stock to a boil, add carrots, cover, and reduce flame to medium-low. Simmer 1 to 2 minutes. Add tofu and tamari soy sauce. Simmer 3 to 5 minutes more. Place several pieces of watercress in individual serving bowls and ladle hot broth over it. Serves 4.

Noodles and Broth
(See chapter 8 on *Grains* for recipe.)

3. *Grain and bean soups:* Any combination of fresh or leftover grains and beans can be made into a delicious soup. Fresh beans and grains will of course require a longer cooking time than soups made with leftovers.
   A. Boiling. To boil, layer the vegetables in a pot. Place the more yin vegetables on the bottom and the more yang ones on top (except for greens which are added later and placed on top). Then add the grains or beans, and enough water just to barely cover everything. Bring to a slow boil, adding more water as the grains or beans expand. You can place a heat deflector underneath to help prevent burning. This is the same method used in boiling beans (see *Beans and Bean Products* chapter), except that instead of boiling away the excess liquid in the

end, we add more to make it soupy. The salt and/or miso or tamari are added after the grain or bean has softened (simmer another 3 to 10 minutes after the seasoning is added). More water can be added if the consistency is too thick.

Millet-Squash Soup

1 cup squash, cubed
½ cup onion, diced
¼ cup carrot, diced
¼ cup celery, diced
1 strip kombu, 3″–4″, soaked, diced
5–6 cups spring water
Sea salt (mild taste)
Scallion or parsley garnish

Use cooking method described above. Layer kombu, onion, celery, squash, carrot, and millet in that order. Then cook as described above.

Hato Mugi (Pearl Barley) Soup

1 cup hato mugi, washed
1 strip kombu, 3″–4″, soaked and diced
½ cup onion, diced
½ cup carrot, diced
¼ cup celery, diced
¼ cup dried daikon, soaked and sliced
½ cup dried tofu, soaked and cubed
1 shiitake mushroom soaked and diced
1 Tbsp. burdock root, diced
5–6 cups water
Sea salt or tamari soy sauce for mild taste
Scallion garnish

Pressure-cook all ingredients for 40 to 45 minutes. Let the pressure come down completely, and uncover. Bring to a boil again, add tamari soy sauce, turn the flame to low, place a heat deflector underneath, and simmer for another 10 minutes. Serves 4.

B. Pressure-cooking. The grains or beans are first pressure-cooked. The cover is then taken off. Then add the salt (especially in the case of beans, as some grain dishes can take salt from the beginning), tamari soy sauce, or miso, and perhaps some vegetables. Now simmer, up to 20 to 30 minutes longer, depending on the dish.

Soybean Stew

1 cup soybeans, soaked 6–8 hours (discard soaking water)
1 strip kombu, 3″–4″, soaked and cubed
2 shiitake mushrooms, soaked and diced
¼ cup celery, diced
¼ cup dried daikon, soaked and sliced
2–3 pieces dried tofu, soaked and cubed
½ cup carrot, diced
¼ cup burdock, cubed
¼ cup lotus root, cubed
½ cup seitan, cubed
5–6 cups water
Tamari soy sauce to taste
Scallion garnish
Optional: grated ginger, 1 pinch per serving bowl

Follow directions as for pressure-cooking soups as explained in the above recipe.

Azuki Bean Soup

1 1″-piece kombu
1 small winter squash, cubed
1 cup dried azuki beans, washed
¼ to ½ tsp. sea salt
1 quart spring water
Sliced scallions or chopped parsley for garnish

Soak the kombu for 5 minutes and slice. Put the beans in a pot and add the water. Bring to a boil, lower the heat, and simmer for 1¼ hours, or until the beans are about 80 percent done. Put the squash cubes in the bottom of another pot, then cover with the beans and kombu. Add the salt and cook for another 20 minutes, or until the squash is soft. Adjust seasoning and garnish with scallions or parsley to serve.

4. *Soup Stocks:* These soup stocks can be used for any of the above types of soups. They are particularly good for the clear, miso, and vegetable soups.

Kombu Soup Stock

1 strip kombu, 3″–6″
5–6 cups spring water

Wipe dust from kombu with a clean, damp cloth. Leave the white powder on. Bring the kombu and water to a boil, simmer about 3 minutes, and remove the kombu. It can be reused for

another stock (boil it longer the next time to get more out of it), added to another dish, or sliced and used in this one.
Other variations:

a) **4 shiitake mushrooms, simmer 5–6 minutes**
b) **2 Tbsps. bonito fish flakes, simmer 3–4 minutes**
c) **Any combination of kombu, shiitake, and bonito**
d) **Odds and ends of vegetables such as onion skins, cabbage cores, roots, tops, and so on. Wash well, boil 5 minutes, and discard or use for compost.**
e) **Other sea vegetables such as wakame and dulse**
f) **Dry-roast grains such as rice, sweet rice, millet, buckwheat, or barley until a nutty fragrance is emitted, and use for stock. Simmer 4–5 minutes.**
g) *Chirimen iriko* **(small, whole dried fish available in natural and Oriental food stores). Boil 2 Tbsps. 3–4 minutes.**
h) **Leftover liquid from boiling vegetables**
i) **Water left over from cooking beans**
j) **Diluted water left over from cooking seitan**

5. *Vegetable Soups:* Vegetable soups and stews are a nice, light, sweet addition to our meals several times per week.

1. They can be prepared simply by boiling various sliced vegetables in water or a prepared soup stock until soft. Then, season either with sea salt, tamari soy sauce, miso, or umeboshi plum. Occasionally, kuzu can be used to thicken vegetable soups for a smooth, creamy consistency.
2. Vegetable soups can also be puréed in a hand food mill, after cooking, for a creamier consistency.
3. Occasionally, if allowed, whole oats, oatmeal, rice or sweet rice may be cooked together with vegetables and then puréed when done, for a heartier, creamy soup.

Squash Soup

1 medium-sized buttercup or butternut squash
4 to 5 cups spring water
1/4 to 1/2 tsp. sea salt
Toasted nori, cut into 1″-squares for garnish
Chopped parsley or sliced scallions for garnish

Wash the squash and remove the skin and seeds. Cut the squash into large chunks to obtain 4 to 5 cups. Put the squash in a pot and add the water and a pinch of sea salt. Bring to a boil. Cover, lower the heat, and simmer until the squash is soft, about 40 minutes to an hour. Pour the squash and cooking water into a hand food mill and puree. Return the puréed squash to the pot, season with the remaining sea salt, and simmer for several minutes. Pour the soup into individual serving bowls and garnish with a few squares of toasted nori and chopped parsley or scallions.

10. Vegetables

As much as possible, get organically grown, chemical-free vegetables. Besides being healthier, they are more delicious. Organic farmers put much care and attention into producing food that benefits both mankind and the planet. Also, avoid dull-colored, limp, yellow-leafed, soft, spotted, or wrinkled items, as they are either too old, spoiled, dried up and/or lacking in vitality.

Choose locally grown produce as often as possible, though in the north during the winter more southern-grown ones will be eaten. Prepackaged items tend to spoil more quickly. Stay away from canned and frozen foods. They have no energy and/or have added salt, sugar, and preservatives, all of which are best avoided. Also, be careful not to buy waxed items.

At home, immediately remove any yellow leaves and spoiled parts of your vegetables before storing them. This helps to preserve the rest for a longer time. When storing vegetables in the refrigerator, keep them in a paper bag; this allows them to absorb extra moisture and thereby retards spoilage. A plastic bag retains water, does not allow your vegetables to breathe, and causes them to grow soggy and spoil more quickly. Keep vegetables separated from fruits for better preservation.

Do not wash vegetables until just before cooking. Any soil left on them helps to keep them fresh longer. When washing vegetables, particularly the leafy greens, it helps to submerge them in a big bowl of water. Gently swish them and then wash each leaf individually. This automatically separates and loosens the sand, soil, and dirt which settles to the bottom of the bowl, as the greens stay afloat. This is much more effective and easier than just trying to rinse them under the tap. Roots can be scrubbed gently with a vegetable brush (*tawashi*) to remove any soil, but make sure to keep the skin on. (Do not peel organic vegetables, as they are not sprayed, or covered with wax. The skins contain many nourishing nutrients.)

To wash leeks, cut them in half lengthwise, and clean out all the dirt trapped between the layers of leaves. The soil usually collects in the section where the colors change from white to green.

Always use cold water when cleaning vegetables as hot water washes out many vitamins and minerals. Wash vegetables quickly. Soaking for any length of time also depletes valuable nutrients.

Within one dish, cut your vegetables uniformly for even cooking.

Within a meal, have a variety of different sizes represented in several dishes—smaller for sautéed items, and bigger chunks for stews, for example.

Save the tops and roots of vegetables. They can be cleaned, chopped very finely, and incorporated into vegetable dishes. You can also leave them uncut and use them in a soup stock. Using the whole plant helps to create a balance in your system.

I recommend the square, Japanese vegetable knives (see *Cookware* chapter) for cutting vegetables. They are very handy, flexible, and easy to use. With these knives, we do not cut straight down, or use them like a saw. Starting with the front tip or edge, gently slide the length of the blade across your vegetables in one smooth stroke. *Important: Always Keep Your Fingertips Curled Underneath So That Your Knuckles Show When You Are Cutting.* This helps to protect the fingers from accidental cuts and slips, and allows a better grip on the vegetable as well.

There are several cutting styles to choose from. Here is a partial listing.

1) Round slices
2) Diagonal slices
3) Triangular shapes
4) Rectangles
5) Half-moons
6) Quarters
7) Matchsticks
8) Shavings
9) Cubing, dicing, and mincing
10) Wedge slices
11) Slicing cabbages
12) Slicing big leafy greens

Fig. 13 Vegetable Cutting Styles

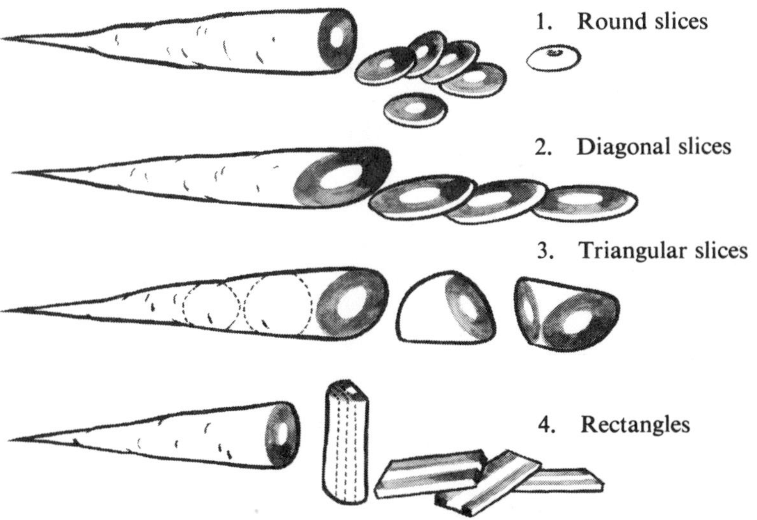

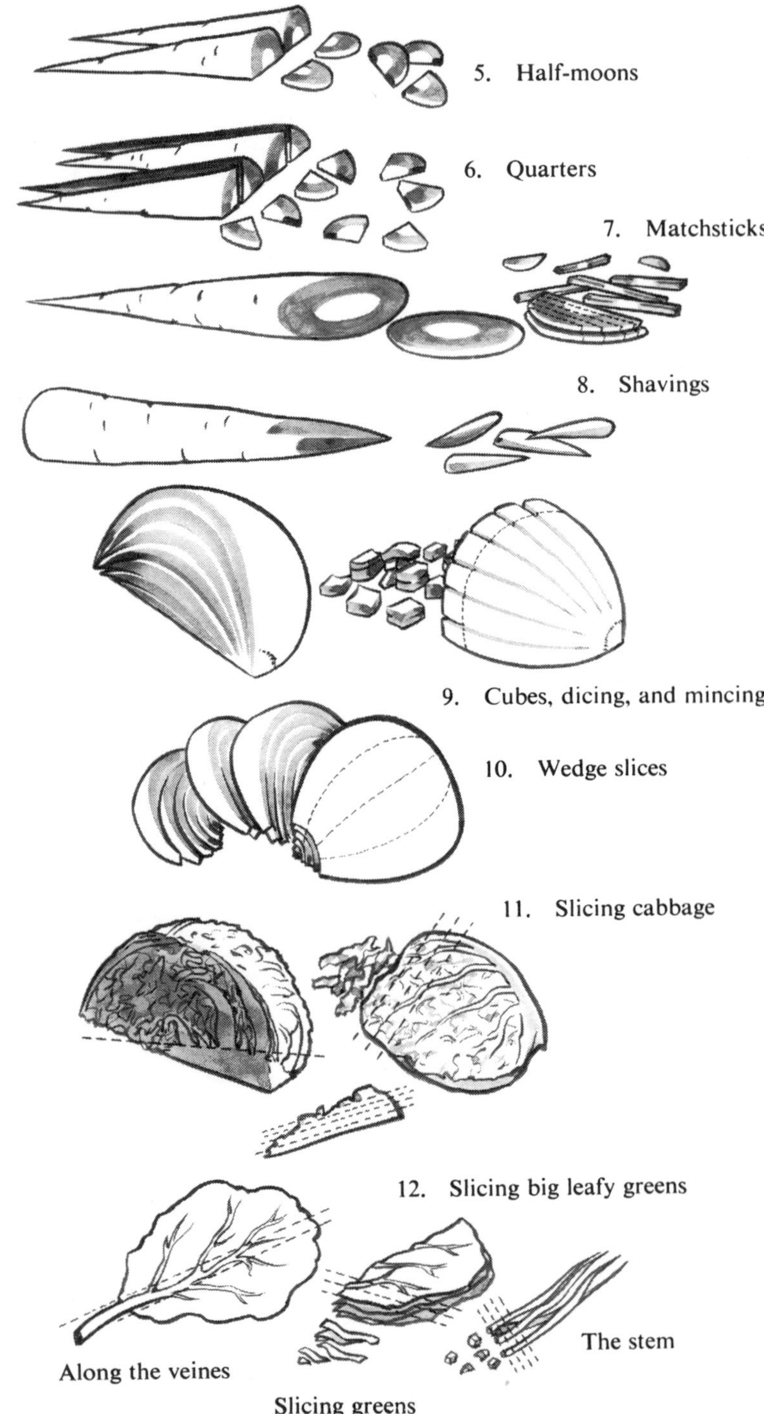
5. Half-moons
6. Quarters
7. Matchsticks
8. Shavings
9. Cubes, dicing, and mincing
10. Wedge slices
11. Slicing cabbage
12. Slicing big leafy greens
The stem
Along the veines
Slicing greens

Include a variety of different kinds of vegetables (roots, greens, ground, and sea vegetables, for example) in a meal as well as an assortment of textures, and colors. Also, use a variety of cooking styles. Here are some of the main methods that we use.

1. *Boiling methods:* There are two main styles of boiling: quick, short-time, and slow, longer-time boiling. Some kind of boiled vegetable can be served at nearly every meal.

   A. Quick boiling (blanching): Blanching is the best way to cook leafy green vegetables. Fill a pot with 1 to 2 inches of water and bring to a boil. Dip in vegetables and take them out quickly. An oil skimmer lifts them easily. Drain the vegetables in a colander. Place a plate underneath to catch excess liquid which can be put back into the pot. Chinese cabbage, broccoli, cauliflower, celery, and others can be used.

   The main point in this style is to cook in as short a time as possible, retaining crispness and bright colors. For example, watercress can be taken out after 15 to 30 seconds. Others take a little longer, in varying degrees, but not much more.

   A pinch of salt in the water helps retain bright colors (but leave it out when cooking bitter vegetables such as watercress and mustard greens, as salt will hold in the bitter flavor).

   Root vegetables can also be cooked in this way but you have to cut them into very thin slices. Boil them for a slightly longer time than you would with greens.

   If you want to boil several different vegetables, do them one by one. Start with the lighter-tasting varieties like the cabbages, and end with more strong-tasting ones like mustard greens, so that the flavor of the latter will not overpower the flavor of the former. Each vegetable's distinct individuality should be maintained.

   You can use the leftover boiling water as a base for a soup. Or you can add some kuzu to it (2 teaspoons for one cup water) to thicken it into a sauce to pour over your vegetables. To do this, first dilute the kuzu in a small amount of cold water. Turn the flame to low under the boiled water and pour the kuzu in. Stir and simmer until the liquid turns clear. Add a little tamari soy sauce or umeboshi paste to taste, and pour this over boiled vegetables.

Boiled Kale

1 small bunch kale

4 cups water
1 pinch sea salt

Bring water and salt to a boil. Thoroughly wash the kale. Boil whole leaves, a few at a time, until they are bright green and just tender. Remove and drain. When cool, cut to desired size.

Boiled Salad

½ Chinese cabbage, separated into leaves
1 bunch watercress
1 onion, cut in thin crescents
1 carrot, cut in matchsticks
1 stalk celery, cut on the diagonal
Spring water
Toasted, ground sesame seeds for garnish

Bring 1 to 2 inches of spring water to a boil with a pinch of sea salt. Boil the vegetables separately in the following order, rinsing each in cold water after they are removed from the pot: Chinese cabbage leaves (1 to 2 minutes); onions (1 minute); carrots (2 minutes); celery (1 minute); watercress (10 seconds).

Slice the cabbage leaves and watercress in thin crosswise slices, mix all vegetables together, adding the toasted sesame seeds and a little rice vinegar, if desired.

B. Slow, longer-time boiling: Slow boiling is basically for root vegetables such as daikon, carrots, onions, lotus root, burdock, and so on, as well as for squash. This style gives a calming but strong and healing energy.

One or two pieces of kombu are usually placed in the bottom of the pot to help prevent the vegetables from burning, to add extra minerals and flavor, and to help harmonize all the ingredients.

The vegetables are then layered on top of the kombu, with the more yin ones on the bottom and the more yang ones on the top. The yin rising energy meets the yang descending energy and the dish is better integrated.

If the vegetables are fairly dry, put in enough water to just cover them. If they are fresh and more watery, cover them only halfway with water. Add a pinch of salt, cover the pot, bring everything to a boil, turn the flame to low, and simmer for about 20 minutes, or until soft. The time depends on the type, quality, and slice sizes of the vegetables used. Do not mix or stir the vegetables. When the vegetables are soft, add some tamari soy sauce for more flavor, and simmer another 5 minutes. Shiitake mushrooms, dried tofu, tempeh, and seitan may also be added to this dish.

Califlower, Carrots, and Leeks

1 small cauliflower, separate the individual flowers
2 carrots, cut into triangular wedges
2 leeks, cut into triangular wedges (as much as possible)
Separate the white stem from the green leaves
1 strip kombu, 3″
1 pinch sea salt
Enough water to half cover the vegetables
***Optional:* Tamari soy sauce to taste**

Place the kombu in the bottom of the pot. Add the white bottom of the leeks, then the carrots, cauliflower, and the leek greens on top. Add water and salt, cover, and follow the above directions, cooking for 12 to 15 minutes, or until all the vegetables are tender. Serves 4 to 5.

Daikon and Kombu

Daikon radish, cut into 1″ rounds
Kombu

Wash kombu and soak until tender. Slice into 1-inch pieces and place them in the bottom of a pot. Add daikon on top and enough water to come to half the height of the vegetables. Add a pinch of sea salt and cook as described in *Slow, Longer-Time Boiling*.

2. *Nishime style:* Nishime is a medicinal form of cooking using a minimal amount of water. For this, either a heavy pot with a heavy lid or some cookware designed for waterless cooking is needed.

Kombu at the bottom of the pot helps to prevent burning as well as adding extra minerals and taste.

Root vegetables such as carrots, daikon, turnips, burdock, lotus root, onions, and hard winter squash (acorn, buttercup, or Hokkaido), cabbage, and shiitake mushrooms are often used. For reproductive disorders, the use of sweet vegetables should be emphasized. The vegetables are layered on top of the kombu from yin to yang (yin on the bottom). Squash dissolves and loses its shape if cooked for a long time, so it can be added a little later on.

To cook, soak a piece of kombu until it is soft, cut it into

1-inch squares, and place it in the bottom of a pot. Add enough water just to cover the kombu if the vegetables are fresh and watery. If they are more dry, or if using burdock or lotus root, add enough water to cover the vegetables halfway. Put in the vegetables and sprinkle a pinch or two of sea salt or a few drops of tamari soy sauce over them.

Cover, set the flame on high until a steam is produced. Then lower the flame and let the vegetables simmer peacefully for 15 to 20 minutes. If water should evaporate during cooking, add a little more to the bottom of the pot if it is necessary to prevent burning.

When all the vegetables have softened, add a few more drops of tamari soy sauce to taste.

Then, replace the cover, and cook over a low flame for 2 to 5 minutes more. After turning off the flame, remove the cover and let the vegetables sit for about 2 minutes. Serve the juice along with the vegetables as it is very delicious.

Squash, Cabbage, Onion, and Kombu

1 pinch sea salt
Water
½ buttercup squash, cut into 2″-chunks
¼ cabbage, cut into 2″-squares
2 onions, quartered
1 strip kombu, 5″, washed, soaked and cut into 2″-pieces
1 pinch sea salt
Tamari soy sauce to taste
Just enough water to cover the kombu

Follow the directions for *Nishimi Style*. Serves 4 to 6.

Daikon/Daikon Greens

Daikon roots and leaves
1 strip kombu, 3″–6″, soaked and sliced
Miso or tamari soy sauce to taste
Enough water to just cover the kombu

Fig. 14 Daikon Radish

Wash and finely slice the daikon roots and leaves. Put the kombu in a pot with enough water to just cover it. Add the roots, cover, and cook with a high steam for 10 minutes or longer. Towards the end, add the leaves, miso or tamari soy sauce to taste and simmer for another 2 to 4 minutes.

Other variations:

1) **Daikon and its greens**
2) **Carrots and their greens (slice greens extra fine)**
3) **Radish and its leaves**
4) **Dandelion root and leaves**

3. *Sautéing:* There are two ways to sauté: with oil or using water as a substitute. When limiting the use of oil, use the water-sautéing method as often as desired. For this method, instead of using oil, as discussed below, simply add a few tablespoons of water to a frying pan, bring to a boil, and simmer the vegetables until they are soft.

When using oil, it is best to use only sesame oil (particularly the dark or roasted variety) and to spread it onto the bottom of a heated pan with a brush, rather than to pour it in. Put oil into a cast-iron skillet, using approximately 1 tablespoon for 8 servings, and heat it up with a medium-high flame. When the oil seems warm, test it by dropping in one slice of a vegetable. If the oil sizzles, it is ready and the rest of the ingredients can be added.

Either add the different kinds of vegetables one by one, starting with those that take the longest time to cook and ending with the faster-cooking ones, or cut the vegetables so that they will cook at the same rate (soft vegetables in larger slices, tougher ones in thinner slices), and layer them from yin to yang (yin on the bottom).

After adding the vegetables, add a pinch or two of sea salt. Salt brings out the natural sweetness, draws out the water, and helps to soften the vegetables quicker (it has the opposite effect on grains and beans and is therefore added later on in their case). Gently stir from time to time (with a wooden spoon or cooking chopsticks) to prevent burning.

After about 5 minutes turn the flame to low, cover (unless working with really watery items such as Chinese cabbage or tofu), and simmer until the vegetables are soft. The time it takes depends on what is being cooked and the size of slices used. It may be necessary to add a little water to avoid burning, especially when cooking with something like burdock. Add a little soy sauce (and some grated ginger if desired) at the end for more flavor, and simmer another 2 to 3 minutes. Uncover and boil away any excess water if there is any.

Any vegetable can be sautéed (cut root vegetables into very thin slices or shavings), as can tofu and tempeh.

Kinpira Carrot and Burdock

(Kinpira is very strengthening and can be used once or twice a week. While generally made with oil, the dish can also be made using the water-sautéing technique described above.)

1 cup shaved burdock
2 cups shaved carrots
Dark sesame oil (optional)
1 pinch sea salt
Tamari soy sauce to taste
½ tsp. juice of grated ginger (optional)
Water, if needed to prevent burning
A few parsley sprigs

Fig. 15 Burdock

Lightly brush sesame oil in a skillet and heat. Place burdock and carrots into the skillet and add a pinch of sea salt. Sauté for 2 to 3 minutes. Add water to lightly cover the bottom of the skillet. Cover and cook until the vegetables are 80 percent done. Add several drops of tamari soy sauce, cover, and cook for several minutes more until the vegetables become tender. Remove the cover and cook until the excess liquid is absorbed. Onions, turnips, and lotus root can be substituted or used together with carrots and burdock.

Sautéed Mustard Greens

1 bunch fresh mustard greens
⅛ tsp. sesame oil or water
½ tsp. tamari soy sauce or to taste
1 tsp. grated ginger

Carefully wash greens and cut to desired shape. Warm a skillet on medium heat and add oil. When oil is hot, add the greens, stir and cover. Cook for about 3 minutes, or until the greens are tender. (Stir once or twice to ensure even cooking.) Remove pan from heat, and mix in tamari soy sauce and ginger. Serves 4 to 6.

Sautéed Vegetables with Tofu

(This type of lighter dish, using some of the "occasional use" vegetables, is very nice for variety and freshness.)

2 celery stalks, cut into thin diagonal slices
2 carrots, cut into thin diagonal slices
1 medium summer squash, cut into thin diagonal slices
1 cake tofu, cut into 1″ cubes
Dark sesame oil or 1–2 Tbsps. water
1 pinch sea salt
Tamari soy sauce to taste
A dash of grated ginger

Heat oil or water in a skillet, sauté tofu, then celery, carrots, and squash. Add sea salt. Do not cover. Boil off any excess liquid. Add tamari soy sauce to taste and simmer another 3 minutes. Add a dash of ginger and serve. Serves 3 to 4.

4. *Pressure-cooking:* When healing, we do not recommend pressure-cooking vegetables. Vegetables cook very quickly compared to grains and beans so we recommend other cooking methods instead. Pressure-cooking is reserved for grains and beans.

5. *Steaming:* Steaming can be used often. To steam, put ½ to 1 inch of cold water in the bottom of a pot, insert a steamer, place vegetables inside, with a pinch of sea salt if desired, cover, and bring the water to a boil. Then steam for 3 to 5 minutes (greens should be steamed only about 3 minutes) or until the vegetables are soft.

   This method is good for any kind of vegetable and is a nice variation on the boiling method. Be careful not to overcook the vegetables. Remove them while they are still crisp and brightly colored.

   Steam each kind of vegetable separately unless they are to be served mixed together and they take the same amount of time to cook. In order for the vegetables to keep their bright color, run them under cold water and don't cover them until they are cool. The leftover water can be used as soup stock or sauce, as with the boiling method. Steaming is also an excellent way to heat up leftovers, especially grains.

Steamed Radishes and Greens

2 bunches radishes with greens intact
1 pinch sea salt
1 tsp. fresh toasted sesame seeds

Bring a pot of water with a steamer basket in it to a full boil. Meanwhile, wash radishes and slice them into ¼-inch-thick rounds. Wash the greens well and cut them into 1-inch pieces. Add the radishes to the steamer, placing the greens on top. Add a pinch of sea salt and cook until the greens and radishes are just tender, but not over-cooked. Remove from pot and toss with sesame seeds, or arrange on a serving dish, and sprinkle on the seeds.

Steamed Squash

2 cups butternut or buttercup squash, sliced thin

Place squash slices in a steamer basket and steam several minutes, until tender.

6. *Salad:* There are three types of salads:
   A. *Boiled salad:* Refer to the section on boiled vegetables for directions and an example. This can be eaten several times a week.

   B. *Pressed salad:* Pressed salad can generally be eaten every two or three days. The vegetables are raw but pressing them with salt helps to yangize them.

   To prepare, cut vegetables into very thin slices, or shred them, and put them in a pickle press with sea salt for one or more hours. Drain off the excess water, wash off the excess salt, and serve. To prepare without a pickle press, put vegetables in a bowl and cover them with a plate. Put a rock or some kind of weight (such as a large glass jar filled with water) on top of the plate and press.

Pressed Salad

2 cups Chinese cabbage, finely shredded
¼ cup celery, sliced thinly on the diagonal
½ cup red radishes, thinly sliced
1 tsp. sea salt

Place all vegetables in a pickle press. Add the sea salt and mix thoroughly. Apply pressure. Press 1½ to 2 hours. Drain off the juice which rises to the surface of the press.

Variations:

1. ½ teaspoon sea salt + ¼ cup brown rice vinegar
2. ¼ cup umeboshi vinegar + ¾ cup water

C. *Regular raw salad:* Persons trying to alleviate such reproductive disorders as low sperm count and sexually transmitted diseases (see *Dietary Adjustments for Infertility and Reproductive Disorders* chapter) should avoid raw salad for a while, perhaps several months. Otherwise, raw salad is recommended about once or twice a week in small quantities, and more often during the hot summer months.

Use the usual salad vegetables such as lettuce, cucumbers, sprouts, carrots, onions, celery, parsley, cabbage, and so on, but avoid peppers, potatoes, tomatoes, eggplants, and mushrooms. Suggestions for additional ingredients include roasted sesame and pumpkin seeds, wholewheat bread croutons, cooked chick-peas, pinto beans, rice, bulgur, couscous, noodles, macaroni, wakame, dried dulse, and cooked hijiki, arame, tofu, tempeh and seitan. Of course, combinations have to be tasteful. Obviously, not all of these ingredients are compatible.

Wakame Salad

1 cup wakame (Wash, soak 10 minutes, boil 2–3 minutes, rinse in cold water, drain, and slice into 1″ pieces.)
½ head iceburg lettuce, cut into bite-sized pieces
1 cucumber, sliced into thin rounds
1 Tbsp. umeboshi paste

Peel cucumber if it is waxed. Cut off the ends and dip them in sea salt. Rub each end piece in a circular motion against the end it was cut from. This helps draw out bitterness from the cucumber. Rinse off sea salt and slice cucumber. Mix wakame, umeboshi paste, lettuce, and cucumber. Serves 5.

Tossed Salad

1 head leafy green lettuce
1 cup alfalfa sprouts
½ cup carrot, cut into very thin matchsticks
1 red onion, sliced into thin rounds
½ pkg. tempeh, cut into cubes, deep-fried or pan-fried, and simmered in kombu stock with tamari soy sauce for ½ hour
1 recipe *Tamari, Ginger, Vinegar Dressing*

Wash lettuce, drain, and cut into bite-sized pieces. Toss all ingredients or arrange artfully on a serving platter. Serve the dressing on the side.

7. *Baking:* Baking foods takes a longer time but it gives strength and extra flavor. It is best to bake once in a while for variety rather than on a daily basis. The method is especially appropriate to the fall and winter seasons as it is a more yang cooking style, and is most suitable to root or round vegetables, such as winter squash. Greens should never be baked.

   Baking can be done with or without oil, using a casserole dish or a cookie sheet covered with foil. If the vegetables are fresh and juicy, it may not be necessary to add water, especially if the sheet or dish is oiled and well-covered. If no oil is used, add just enough water to cover the cooking surface. More water may be needed if the vegetables are tough or a bit dried out. Adding a pinch of salt helps to draw out water from the vegetables.

   The vegetables should be cooked at 350° to 375°F. for approximately 45 to 50 minutes, or until they are soft.

   Squash can be baked whole and uncovered, on an oiled cookie sheet, with a stuffing, or sliced in halves or chunks. If halved, place the halves on a cookie sheet uncovered, with the inside facing down.

   Baked Stuffed Squash

   1–2 acorn squash
   1 cup millet, pressure-cooked with 1½ cups spring water for 15 minutes, or boiled for 25 minutes with 2 cups water
   ¼ cup onions, diced
   ¼ cup carrots, diced
   ⅛ cup celery, diced
   1 sliced mushroom
   ¾–1 cup chopped seitan

   Combine the millet, onions, carrots, celery, mushroom, and seitan. Cut the tops off the squash and scoop out the seeds. Fill the squash with the millet mixture (if it is very dry, moisten this mixture with about ½ cup of seitan juice or spring water). Place the squash in a baking dish in which a small amount of spring water has been added. Cover the dish with foil and bake at 350°F. approximately 35 to 40 minutes or until the squash is tender.

8. *Pickles:* Pickles are an extremely important addition to the diet. Have a small amount on the side at every meal or at least once

a day, and eat them with grains. They aid in digestion, strengthen the intestinal flora, stimulate appetite, and add zest to the meal. If the pickles are very salty, rinse them quickly before serving or, if necessary, soak them in cold water for 5 minutes.

Always use fresh, firm, and crisp vegetables for making pickles. Also, it is imperative that the vegetables, containers, and anything else used for pickling, be thoroughly cleaned. This is done to prevent any unknown substances interacting with the pickling process. For tougher vegetables, it is helpful to quickly blanch them in boiling water before pickling them.

Pickling time ranges from a couple of hours to several months. The main factors influencing pickling time are the size of vegetables and the amount of salt used. Small, thinly sliced pieces can be pickled very quickly whereas large, thick, or whole pieces take a long time. Long-time pickling requires more salt to prevent spoiling. Vegetables can be dipped in hot boiling water before pickling, if desired, especially with largely sliced and/or hard vegetables. This removes the raw flavor and brings out a sweeter taste.

Experimentation may be needed to get the feel of the right amount of salt to use. If the vegetables spoil before they pickle, and/or not much water comes out (for methods that require that it does), then there is not enough salt. If too much salt is added, the pickles will become too salty and any other flavor that the vegetables may have had will be covered up. To remove excess salt, rinse or soak pickles for a little while before serving them.

If mold starts to form anywhere, remove it immediately so that the rest of the contents will not be affected.

Cover the container with a cheesecloth. This helps to keep dirt and dust out of the pickles while letting the air circulate and enabling the vegetables to breathe. (Do not cover with an airtight lid.)

There are four main types of pickling methods that we usually use.

1. *Pressed pickles:* Pressed pickles can be made quickly, in a couple of hours, or over several weeks.

   A. *Quick pickles:* When pickling for a few hours up to a day or two, a pickle press can be used. But since most presses are made of plastic, it is not safe to use them for a longer period of time as the poisonous toxic substances in them will start to seep into the vegetables. An alternative is to take a small glass bowl and find a saucer that fits into it. It should cover the inside as much as possible but still remain loose so that water can escape over the sides. For a weight, use a glass jar full of water, grains, or beans, or some clean stones.

Soft, watery vegetables like thinly sliced cucumbers and very thin matchstick daikon strips can be done in 2 to 3 hours. Other pickles can be made in the morning and be either eaten for dinner or left for 2 to 3 days longer. Some (like harder, less watery vegetables like turnips) may need the extra days. Again, pickling time depends on the size and moisture content of the pieces.

Vegetables have to be cut into really thin slices or shredded for quick pickling. (An exception is mustard greens which can be made whole and cut when ready to serve. Mix the salt in really well and wait 2 to 3 days.) Chinese cabbage, red and white cabbage, daikon and its greens, turnip and its greens, celery, radishes, onions, cucumbers, and bok choy are good to use. For best results, use only one kind of vegetable at a time. Add a strip of kombu (perhaps 3 to 6 inches long for two cups of vegetables) for extra minerals and a different flavor. Soak the kombu until it is soft, slice it into thin strips, and put it underneath the vegetables. Grated ginger can be added if desired.

For 2 cups of vegetables add about 1 to 2 teaspoons of salt. Mix them together thoroughly. The salt can be substituted with 2 to 4 tablespoons of umeboshi vinegar, paste, or plums and/or shiso leaves. You can also use 2 to 4 tablespoons of soy sauce. Water will start to rise above the saucer or pressure plate. If there is a lot, remove a little, but always leave some of it covering the plate. Cover with a cheesecloth (not necessary if using a press, of course) and wait till it is all done.

Onion Pickles

2 cups thinly sliced onions
2–4 Tbsp. tamari soy sauce

Pickle the onions in soy sauce following the above directions. If the onions were cut thinly, they will be done in 2 hours. You can also eat them the next day.

B. *Longer-time pressed pickles:* A wooden keg or ceramic crock are good containers to use for this. A heavy stone or large jar filled with water is placed on top of a plate or a wooden disc, which fits inside, for pressure. Cover the whole thing with a cheesecloth and place in a cool, dark place. Check regularly for mold and remove it immediately if any appears. Sauerkraut is made this way. Below is a sample recipe.

Pressed Daikon Pickles

4–5 daikon radish
½ cup sea salt

Wash, dry completely and cut the daikon into several lengthwise strips. Place a layer of salt in a crock or wooden keg. Then add a layer of daikon. Then a layer of salt. Alternate until all the daikon is used. Salt should be the last layer. Place a weight on top, cover with a cheesecloth, and press for 1 to 2 weeks. Chinese cabbage, carrots, turnips, daikon greens, and so on can all be pickled this way.

2. *Brine pickles:* To make brine pickles, tightly stuff some vegetables into a glass jar. Boil some kind of a brine mixture (see below), let it cool, and then pour it into the jar, filling it up. Cover the top with cheesecloth which is fastened down with a rubber band, and pickle for several days. When done, store pickles in a refrigerator. This is how dill pickles are made. A variety of vegetables can be used, including cucumbers, onions, turnips, rutabagas, daikon, carrots, broccoli, cauliflower, cabbages, greens, and so on.

There are several kinds of brine that can be used, examples of which are presented below. A soup stock can be used if desired. For extra flavor, add ginger, kombu, shiitake mushrooms, lemon juice and rinds, shiso leaves, grated raw apple, and so on. Some *ame* rice syrup can be boiled and dissolved into the brine, especially in the case of tamari-based pickles, as it gives a delicious sweet taste.

Onion Cucumber Pickles (Salt-based Brine)

3 lbs. pickling cucumbers
2 onions, quartered
12 cups spring water
¼–⅓ cup sea salt

Bring water and salt to a boil. Turn flame to medium-low and simmer until all the salt has dissolved. Allow this mixture to cool. Wash and place cucumbers and onions into a large glass jar or crock. Pour the cooled brine in, filling the container to the top. Cover with a cheesecloth and keep in a cool, dark place for 5 to 10 days. When pickles are done, store them in the refrigerator.

Turnip Pickles

4 turnips, sliced very thinly, lengthwise
1½ tsps. sea salt
2 tsps. chopped lemon peel

Mix all ingredients together by hand. Place the turnips in a bowl, cover, and leave overnight. Rinse the pickles before eating them. These can be refrigerated for up to one week.

Cauliflower and Radish Pickles (Umeboshi-based Brine)

Enough cauliflower to fill a glass quart jar
5 radishes, cut in half
2 cups water
1 cup umeboshi vinegar
5 shiso leaves

Place cauliflower and radishes into a jar. Mix the water, umeboshi vinegar, and shiso leaves together and pour over vegetables. Cover with a cheesecloth and let set for 3 to 4 days.

3. *Miso pickles:* Miso pickles are especially helpful for recovering good digestive strength. They are simple to make. Just quickly blanch vegetables in boiling water, then submerge and surround them totally in miso. This is used for root vegetables such as carrots, burdock, daikon, turnips, parsnips, and ginger. Broccoli stems make great pickles as well. Greens are too watery.

   The vegetables have to be dried out until they can be bent like rubber before being added to the miso. Otherwise, the miso will get too watery and the pickling won't work.

   Pickling time depends on the vegetables being used and the size of the slices. Very thin ones can pickle in 3 to 4 days, up to a week. Whole vegetables with slits in their sides can take 1 to 2 weeks, thick slices about 3 months, and whole vegetables (unslitted) can be left in the miso up to a year. Just make sure they are totally submerged (top, bottom, and sides). Pressure is not needed when making miso pickles.

   When the pickles are done, just take them out, rinse them off, slice, and eat them.

Broccoli Stem Miso Pickles

Broccoli stems
A container of miso

Peel leftover broccoli stems unless the skins are soft, quickly blanch them in boiling water, and submerge them into the miso for 1 to 2 weeks, depending on how thick they are. You can leave the skins on if you like. The pickling time will be much longer then, maybe a month or more. Cover with a cheesecloth and keep in a cool, dark place until they are done.

4. *Bran pickles:* Bran pickling uses a mixture of bran (rice or wheat) or rice flour, and sea salt. Like miso pickles, bran pickles are especially good for weak intestines.

Quickly dry-roast the bran or flour in a skillet over a medium-low flame until a nutty fragrance is emitted. Remove from the skillet and allow it to cool.

Firm, root vegetables pickle best, but you can also use greens. The vegetables should all be dried before you use them. A few hours under the sun works nicely. Daikon, carrots, and parsnips are best when dried longer (several days), until they bend like rubber.

A ceramic crock or wooden keg again are the best containers to use. Cover the pickles with a cheesecloth and keep in a cool, dark place.

There are two ways to make bran pickles.

A. *Bran pickles A:* Boil some salt and water, let it cool off, place in a crock or keg, and thoroughly mix in the roasted bran or flour to form a paste. Take your dried vegetables and totally submerge them into this paste making sure that the vegetables are not touching each other. Pack this whole thing down until it is firm and solid. Cover with a cheesecloth.

If you slice the vegetables into fairly small pieces they will be done in a week or two. You can also leave them whole. Whole root vegetables can take as long as 3 to 5 months to pickle. Add more salt if you want to pickle for a long time. (Whole leaves take only a couple of weeks.)

As you remove your finished pickles, you can keep adding new vegetables. When you do, add more bran and salt. Mix the paste once in a while. If kept well, you can use this paste for years as you add and subtract vegetables from it.

Short-Time Paste Proportions (1–2 Weeks)

10–12 cups bran or rice flour
$\frac{1}{8}$–$\frac{1}{4}$ cup sea salt
3–5 cups water

Longer-Time Paste Proportions (Up to 3–5 Months)

10–12 cups bran or rice flour
1$\frac{1}{2}$–2 cups sea salt
3–5 cups water

B. *Bran pickles B:* This method is made by alternating layers of vegetables with layers of the bran and sea salt mixture.

Mix roasted bran with sea salt and cover the bottom of a crock or keg. Then, add a layer of dried vegetables. Add another layer of bran and salt. Keep alternating. The last layer should be bran. Insert a plate or a wooden disc into the crock on top of the mixture, place a heavy weight on top of the plate, and press the whole thing. The plate or disc should be loose fitting but wide enough to cover the contents as much as possible. A clean stone or a jar filled with water can be used as a weight. Cover with a cheesecloth and put in a cool, dark place. When water begins to rise, lighten the weight. When pickles are done, rinse off the bran, slice, and eat.

Just as in *Bran pickles A*, you can either slice the vegetables into fairly small pieces or leave them whole. As before, whole pieces take a much longer time to pickle and require more salt.

- **Short-Time Proportions (1–2 Weeks)**

10–12 cups bran or rice flour
$\frac{1}{8}$–$\frac{1}{4}$ cups sea salt

- **Longer-Time Proportions (3–5 Months)**

10–12 cups bran or rice flour
1$\frac{1}{2}$–2 cups sea salt

Chinese Cabbage Bran Pickles

2 heads Chinese cabbage
Bran & salt using shorter-time proportions

Separate the individual leaves from the body of the cabbage. Dry the leaves for two days, preferably under the sun. Make alternating layers of cabbage with sea salt (the bottom and top layers should be salt) and place a plate and heavy weight on top. Water should rise to the level of the plate in 10 hours. If not, add more weight and/or a little more salt.

When the water has risen, drain it out thoroughly. Then relayer the cabbage alternating it with the bran. (The bottom and top layers should be bran.) Replace the weight.

The pickles should be ready in a week. When done, wash out the bran, slice, and serve. (The reason for draining out the water first is to produce a less salty and more sweet-tasting pickle. Also, the Chinese cabbage is a pretty watery vegetable. Other vegetables can be layered in one step, using the bran the first time around, as mentioned before this recipe.)

11. Beans and Bean products

Beans are high in protein and are a delicious addition to your diet. It is important not to overeat beans, to chew them very well, and to cook them thoroughly, otherwise they can cause gas, intestinal problems, and a sluggish condition. Beans should always be a side dish, not compromising more than 15 percent of the meal. As they make a heavier dish, beans are more appropriate for supper, somewhat less often for lunch, and generally not for breakfast.

Azuki beans, chick-peas, lentils, and black soybeans are the most yang beans and the best ones to use on a regular basis. Use these beans, and/or bean products such as tofu and tempeh, about three to six times a week (but in small quantities) when healing. Other beans such as pintos, kidneys, black beans, and red lentils can be eaten occasionally, about once a week or less during the healing process, or may be avoided altogether for several months. Soybeans (which are full of protein) need particular attention so that they are cooked thoroughly. They are delicious in combination with vegetables. They can also be eaten in the form of tofu, tempeh, natto, miso, and tamari soy sauce.

When washing beans, first spread them out a little at a time and remove stones or anything else that may be mixed in. Then place the beans in a bowl, cover them with water, and stir. Rinse off any dust that may rise to the surface. Repeat this about 3 times or until the water becomes clear. When lifting beans out of the water into a strainer or colander to drain, leave out any heavy dust or residue that remains in the bottom of the bowl.

Except for red and green lentils, beans may be soaked for a few hours or overnight prior to cooking. This softens them and helps to cook them quicker. Azuki beans need only a few hours of soaking, and from time to time may be cooked without soaking, particularly when trying to strengthen an overly yin condition. Soaking is preferred for pinto and kidney beans for more digestibility. Chick-peas and soybeans should always be soaked, as they are particularly tough. Use the soaking water as part of the cooking liquid.

Salt is to be added towards the end of the cooking process after the beans have already softened, otherwise they will remain hard. Placing a piece of kombu on the bottom of the pot also helps to soften them, and adds additional minerals and flavor.

1. *Boiling:* This is the method I prefer the most as it cooks the beans gently, slowly, and thoroughly. Beans turn out really delicious and much sweeter when boiled.

Soak the beans for a few hours or overnight (not necessary for lentils and split peas). Place an optional piece of kombu on the bottom of a pot, then your choice of optional vegetables and finally the beans on top. Add enough water to just cover the beans. Place a drop top inside the pot to sit directly on the beans. This top should be loose fitting to let steam escape on the sides but large enough to cover the inside of the pot as much as possible.

As the beans expand, slowly and gently pour more *cold* water down the sides of the pot from time to time, always enough to just cover them. The sudden cold water helps the beans to soften more quickly. Bring this to a boil over a medium flame.

Then, turn the flame to medium-low and let it simmer for 45 minutes to an hour or so, continuing to add cold water once in a while. Watch closely to see when more water is needed to prevent burning. Do not stir or mix at all, letting the cooking go on undisturbed. This makes for a tastier dish.

When the beans are 70 percent done, add salt and/or miso or tamari soy sauce, remove the drop top, and simmer for another 10 to 20 minutes, or until the beans are completely soft, boiling away any excess liquid.

Basic Black Soybeans

2 cups black soybeans
6 cups cold spring water
¼ tsp. sea salt
1¼–1½ Tbsps. tamari soy sauce

Wash the beans with cold water very quickly and put them in a bowl. Cover with about 6 cups of water. Add sea salt and let the beans soak for several hours or overnight.

Put the beans in a pot with the salted soaking water and bring to a boil. Reduce the heat to medium-low and simmer until the beans are about 90 percent done. During the simmering, add water when necessary as the liquid evaporates. As the beans cook, skim off and discard any skins that float to the surface, as well as any gray foam that surfaces.

When the beans are about 90 percent done, add the tamari soy sauce. Shake the pot gently up and down to evenly coat the beans with the juice and tamari. Do not mix with a spoon.

Shaking gives the skins a very shiny black appearance. Cook until almost all the remaining liquid has evaporated.

Total cooking time for this dish is about 2½ to 3 hours.

Azuki Beans, Squash, and Kombu

1 cup azuki beans
1 piece kombu, 3″ long
2 cups buttercup or acorn squash or Hokkaido pumpkin
Spring water
2 pinches sea salt

Wash and soak the azuki beans with the kombu for 4 to 5 hours. Remove the kombu and chop it into small squares. Place the kombu in the bottom of a pot and add the squash which has been cut into cubes. Cover the squash with the beans, and add water to just cover the squash layer.

Do not cover the beans at the beginning. Place the bean mixture over low heat and bring to a boil slowly. Cover after about 10 to 15 minutes. Cook until the beans are 70 to 80 percent done, about 1 hour or more.

The water will evaporate as the beans expand, so add cold water occasionally to keep the water level constant. Add sea salt and cook until the beans are done and most of the liquid has evaporated, approximately 15 to 30 minutes more. Transfer to a serving bowl and serve.

Azuki Beans and Wheat Berries

2 cups azuki beans, soaked 6–8 hours
¼–½ cup wheat berries, soaked 6–8 hours
4–5 cups water (include soaking water)
¼–½ tsp. sea salt
1 strip kombu, 6″–8″, soaked and diced

Place azuki, wheat, kombu, and water in a pressure cooker.

2. *Pressure-cooking:* This is the best method for chick-peas as they are extremely hard and tough. Azuki, pinto, and kidney beans can also be pressure-cooked.

   Red and green lentils, split peas, and black and white soybeans may clog the pressure gauge of the pressure cooker and cause a possible explosion, so it is best to boil them. In the case of the lentils and split peas, it does not matter much as they soften very quickly anyway. With soybeans, there are three things you can do to make them safer for pressure-cooking.

A. Boil the (presoaked) soybeans and skim off all the foam that rises to the top. When no more foam appears (maybe in a half hour), place them in a pressure cooker and cook till done.

B. Dry-roast the soybeans before pressure-cooking them. Combining black soybeans with rice or another grain, in addition to the roasting, helps even further.

C. Soak black soybeans for several hours or overnight with ⅛ teaspoon of sea salt for every cup of beans. This helps to prevent the skins from coming off and clogging the gauge.

Pressure-cook 40 to 45 minutes. Bring pressure down, season with sea salt, and cook another 10 to 15 minutes.

Variations:

1. Azuki beans and chestnuts
2. Azuki with raisins and rice syrup
3. Azuki with lotus seeds
4. Azuki with carrots and onions
5. Azuki with dates

3. *Baking:* Baking is a delicious way to cook beans in the winter as it is very hearty.

This method takes the longest time to prepare but the results are well worth the wait. Pintos, kidneys, and soybeans yield well to baking.

To prepare, first place the presoaked beans in a pot on top of the stove, adding 4 to 5 cups of water for every cup of beans. Bring this to a boil, and boil for 15 to 20 minutes to loosen the bean skins.

Then, pour the beans and liquid into a baking pot. (You can place an optional piece of kombu underneath.) Cover, place in the oven, and bake at 350°F., adding more water from time to time as needed. They may be done in about 3 to 4 hours, depending on the type of beans used.

You may add some vegetables halfway through. The salt and/or tamari or miso should be added after the beans have become soft and creamy. After adding the salt, you can take the cover off and let the beans brown a bit. Then, remove from the stove and serve.

Bean Products:

While healing, it is best not to overconsume bean products. Have a small amount 2 to 3 times a week, frequently substituting dried for fresh tofu during the healing process.

1. Tofu or soybean curd comes in two forms, fresh and dried. The fresh tofu available in Oriental shops is usually prepared using a modern chemicalized curdling agent and it is best to buy natural tofu curdled with *nigari* (which comes from sea salt). This is available in natural food stores, and now in many supermarkets. Dried tofu is more strengthening and can be kept indefinitely. Fresh tofu is more yin and should always be cooked.

   a) *Fresh tofu:* After buying fresh tofu, open the package and store the tofu in the refrigerator submerged in fresh water (throw out the water it came in). Before cooking with it, very quickly rinse the tofu under the tap.

   Tofu cooks very quickly and can be boiled, steamed, baked or broiled, sautéed or pan-fried. It is actually done as soon as it is heated up. It can be prepared in many ways.

   When boiling tofu, cut it into cubes, put it into boiling water, and when it rises to the top, it is finished. Add it to soup towards the end of preparation. For miso soup, put in the tofu just before adding the miso.

   To steam tofu cut it into smaller cubes and steam until it becomes hot.

   When sautéing with tofu, do not add any extra water as a lot will come out of the tofu. To remove this excess liquid place the whole cube on a wooden cutting board and prop the board up on one end. Put another cutting board, a heavy plate, or a weight on top of the tofu and let it drain for one hour.

Fig. 16 Tofu

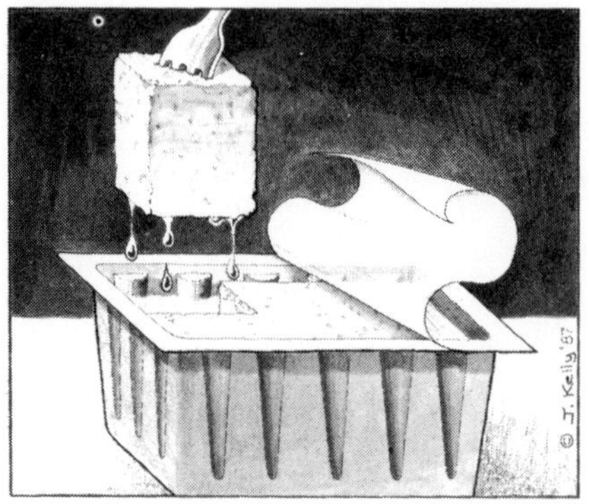

When pan-frying, baking, or broiling, cut the tofu into slabs, heat a thin layer of oil or water in a skillet or baking/broiling sheet, add the tofu and cook the slices until they brown or become hot. This only takes a few minutes so be careful not to burn them. For variety, before or after cooking, spread, dip, or marinate each slice of tofu in one of several sauces or dips including: 1) grated ginger and tamari soy sauce, 2) dry-roasted sesame seeds with tamari soy sauce, 3) diluted miso and chopped onions or scallions.

Boiled Tofu with Chinese Cabbage and Carrots

1 cake tofu
3–5 Chinese cabbage leaves cut into 1″ slices
1 carrot cut into very thin slices
2–3 cups water
1 strip kombu, 3″–6″
1 Tbsp. tamari soy sauce
2–3 chopped scallions
1 tsp. grated ginger

Make a kombu stock by boiling, then simmering kombu in water for 3 to 5 minutes. Remove kombu and save for another use. Place carrots, Chinese cabbage, and tofu into separate sections of the pot and boil them for a few minutes until they are done. Make a dip by taking 1 tablespoon of the stock and mixing in the tamari soy sauce, scallions, and ginger. Serves 2 to 3.

Pickled Tofu
(An unusual but absolutely delicious dish, very similar in taste to cheese.)

1 cake firm tofu
Enough miso to coat tofu

Completely cover tofu with a ¼-inch layer of miso. Let this sit (refrigerate in summer) for 1 to 3 days. The longer the tofu pickles, the more miso-flavored and salty it will become. Scrape off miso and save for another use. Thoroughly rinse tofu before serving. You can also cook tofu before pickling. *Fair Warning:* Only make a small amount at a time, it is very easy to over eat.

b) *Dried tofu:* Dried tofu can be bought at natural or Oriental food stores. It looks like thin, lightly yellow, rectangular wafers.

To cook, first soak it in water until it softens. Then cut it into any desired size or leave it whole. This can be combined with vegetables and treated like one of them. It should be boiled at least 15 minutes. Dried tofu can also be pressure-cooked and used in soups and stews.

Dried Tofu, Carrots, and Onions

2 Tbsps. dark sesame oil (optional)
1 cup onions, sliced into half-moons
1 cup carrots, cut into matchsticks
Spring water
1 cup dried tofu, soaked and sliced
2 tsps. tamari soy sauce

Heat the sesame oil in a frying pan and add the onions. (Or water-sauté the onions in a small amount of spring water.) Add the carrots and enough water to cover the bottom of the pan. Add the sliced tofu and sauté for 1 to 2 minutes. Bring to a boil. Add a little tamari soy sauce. Reduce the heat to low and cover.

Simmer for several minutes, or until the carrots and onions are done. Season with a little more tamari soy sauce, mix and sauté until all the liquid has evaporated. Transfer to a serving bowl and serve.

2. *Tempeh:* Tempeh is a fermented soy product used in Indonesia and available in most natural food stores. It is energizing and full of protein. Store it in the refrigerator.

   Tempeh can be cooked from a few minutes to 30 minutes or more. The longer it is cooked, the more digestible and smoother-tasting it becomes.

   In boiling, steaming, pressure-cooking, baking, and sautéing

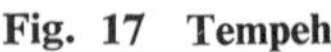
Fig. 17 Tempeh

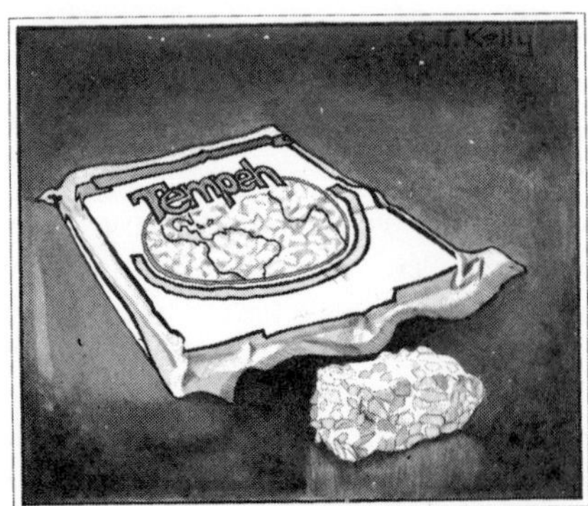

with vegetables, pan- or deep-fry the tempeh beforehand, to make the dish especially delicious. Tempeh can be deep-fried without any batter or covering. Unlike fresh tofu, add it to dishes in the beginning of the cooking preparation.

Boiled Tempeh and Leeks

8 oz. pkg. tempeh, cubed
2 leeks, sliced
Water
Tamari soy sauce to taste

Place tempeh in a skillet and cover with water. Bring to a boil, cover, and reduce flame to medium-low. Simmer 20 to 30 minutes. Add leeks and several drops of tamari soy sauce. Cover and simmer 3 to 4 minutes, or until leeks are done. Remove cover and cook off all liquid. Mix and serve.
Serves 4.

3. *Natto:* Natto is a stringy, fermented, soybean product. At first, the smell may be unpleasant to some individuals. However, once a taste is acquired for natto, many people cannot get enough of it.

Natto is rich in protein and vitamin B_{12}; it imparts vitality and is easily digested and assimilated. It can be purchased at natural or Oriental food stores. Natto generally comes frozen; thaw it by leaving it in the refrigerator for a day, or at room temperature for a few hours.

To serve, stir in one or more of the following ingredients: 1) grated daikon, 2) grated ginger, 3) chopped scallions, or 4) diced raw onions with the addition of either tamari soy sauce, umeboshi paste, or sauerkraut. Pieces of nori may also be mixed in. These combinations may be eaten on top of rice or other grains as a condiment, or in miso soup.

Occasionally, natto may be spooned into miso soup for variety.

12. Sea Vegetables

Sea vegetables are an important and integral part of the macrobiotic diet. They help purify and strengthen the bloodstream and strengthen the intestines, digestive system, liver, pancreas, sexual organs, and enhance mental clarity and awareness. They also help promote beautiful skin and hair. Sea vegetables can be consumed every day in some form, whatever one's condition. They supply calcium, iron, protein, iodine, and vitamins A, B_{12}, and C, as well as various other minerals.

Many people used to (and some still do) cringe at the thought of eating sea vegetables, and considered it an esoteric Oriental food. However, sea vegetables were consumed traditionally by people all over the world including the Celtics, Vikings, Russians, coastal Africans, Mediterranean peoples, North and South American Indians, native Australians, and the early New England settlers (dulse and kombu in their case), as well as people in the Far East. Some varieties may take a while to acquire a taste for, but it is well worth the effort for all the benefits that they bestow.

Sea vegetables are purchased dried (from natural food stores) and can be kept for quite a while before using. They are easily stored. Any shady, dry place will do.

Several varieties of sea vegetables are now available. Kombu is more tough and may take several hours of cooking, unless pressure-cooked, to completely soften. Dulse, on the other hand, can be eaten raw, or like nori, just toasted for a few seconds.

Wash sea vegetables very quickly to retain as much of their nutrients as possible. Submerge hijiki, wakame, and arame in water, rinse off any dust that floats to the top, and lift them out of the water, leaving behind any sand or stones that sit at the bottom. (Arame will probably be pretty clean already as it has been shredded.)

To clean kombu, brush off any dirt or dust with a dry or damp towel. Leave the white-colored substance (which consists of salt and complex sugars) on the surface of the kombu, as it contributes to the flavor and nutritional value. Dulse does not need to be washed in water, but check it very carefully for hidden shells, stones, and tiny fish. Nori and agar-agar should not be washed.

1. *Arame and hijiki:* Arame comes shredded and has a very delicious but mild flavor. Hijiki is naturally stringy and looks like a thicker, darker arame. It also has a richer taste. Hijiki should be soaked

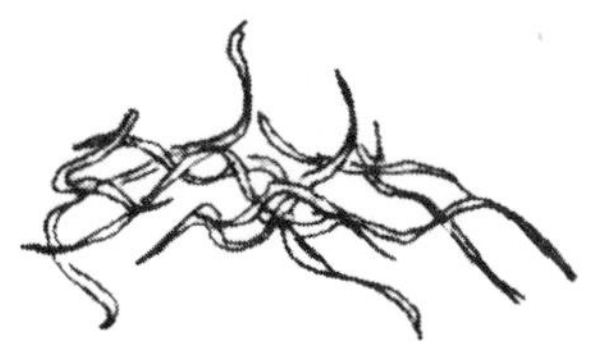

Fig. 18 Dried Arame

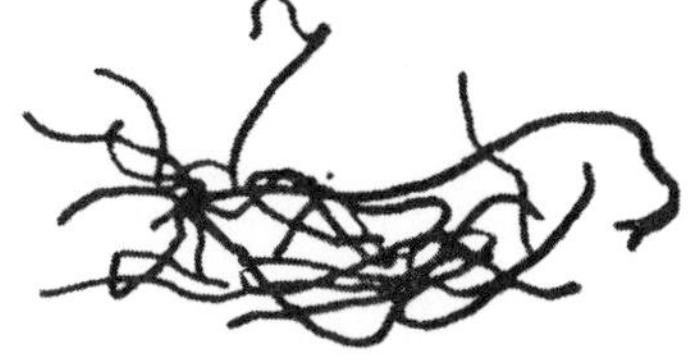

Fig. 19 Dried Hijiki

for 3 to 5 minutes until it expands a bit. Remember that it finally becomes 3 to 5 times larger, so be careful not to use more than you need. It is not necessary to soak arame, just quickly rinse it once in cold water.

Arame and hijiki are cooked the same way, though hijiki takes a longer time, and one can be substituted for the other. They combine really well with root vegetables or with seitan, tofu, tempeh, and fresh corn, as well as other ingredients. They are generally sautéed or just simmered with a small amount of water. It is nice occasionally to sauté the vegetables first before adding the sea vegetable.

Arame with Dried Tofu and Carrots

1 oz. dried arame
2 pieces dried tofu, soaked and cubed
Spring water
1 cup carrots, cut into matchsticks
2 tsps. tamari soy sauce
½ Tbsp. mirin

Wash the arame and drain in a colander. Heat enough spring water to just cover the bottom of a skillet. Add the arame and carrots and sauté 1 to 2 minutes.

Add the dried tofu and enough water to cover the arame and carrots. Add a little tamari soy sauce. Bring to a boil, cover, and reduce the heat to low. Simmer for 40 to 45 minutes. Season with a little more tamari soy sauce and the mirin, and simmer for 10 to 15 minutes longer. When nearly all the liquid has evaporated, mix and serve.

Hijiki with Carrots and Lotus Root

1 oz. hijiki
1 cup carrots, cut into thin matchsticks
¾ cup lotus root, sliced into thin half-moons
Water

Tamari soy sauce
Optional: **¼ tsp. dark sesame oil**

Wash and drain hijiki. (If it is still tough, it can be soaked for 3 to 5 minutes. The soaking water can be used in cooking if it is not too salty.) Heat a skillet with a small amount of oil (you can just brush the bottom) or water. Sauté the hijiki and carrots for 2 to 3 minutes. Add water to half the height of the ingredients. Layer lotus root on top and add a small amount of tamari soy sauce. Cover, bring to a boil, and simmer for 35 to 40 minutes. Add more tamari to taste if desired, and continue to cook for 20 minutes more or until liquid evaporates.

2. *Kombu:* Kombu comes in thick, flat strips which may be anywhere from 3 to 18 inches long. There are recipes throughout this cookbook using kombu, as it enhances the flavor of grains, beans, and vegetable dishes, helping them to soften and/or effectively combining and synthesizing all the ingredients into a whole. It also makes an excellent soup stock. (See *Soup* chapter.) In many cases, kombu is used as an accessory to other ingredients in a dish, but it can be used as a vegetable in its own right. Its texture tends to be tough, so pressure-cooking is often the preferred cooking method, although it can also be boiled.

   Kombu needs to be soaked before slicing. It doubles in size, so be careful how much is used. Soak only until it becomes soft enough to cut. Otherwise, it becomes slippery and slicing will be difficult.

Fig. 20 Kombu

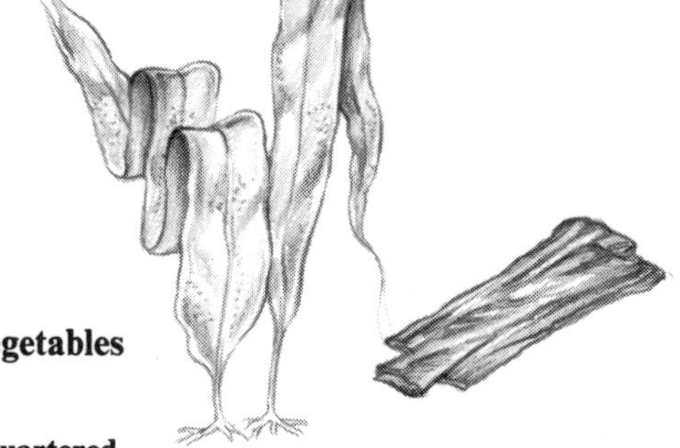

Baked Kombu and Vegetables

1 strip kombu, 3″
2 onions, peeled and quartered
2 carrots, cut into triangular shapes
½ cabbage, sliced into ½″ strips
½ cup spring water
1½ Tbsps. tamari soy sauce

Wash and soak the kombu and put it in a baking dish. Arrange the onions in one side of the dish, the carrots in the center, and the cabbage at the other side, being sure to keep the vegetables separated. Pour the water into a dish and add the tamari soy sauce. Cover and bake in a preheated 375°F. oven for 30 to 40 minutes, or until all the ingredients are tender.

3. *Wakame:* Wakame is a thin, leafy type of sea vegetable and cooks quickly. It can be used in any recipe that calls for kombu. As is kombu, wakame is excellent in grains, beans, vegetable dishes, and soups.

Wakame should be soaked before being sliced. If the soaking water is a bit salty, save it for soups, grains, or bean dishes, where it will be more diluted. Or, to use some of the flavor that went into the liquid for the wakame dish, combine a portion of it with fresh water.

The vein portion takes a longer time to cook. Slice that part fairly thin so that it will be finished when the softer leafy sections (which should be sliced into larger pieces) are.

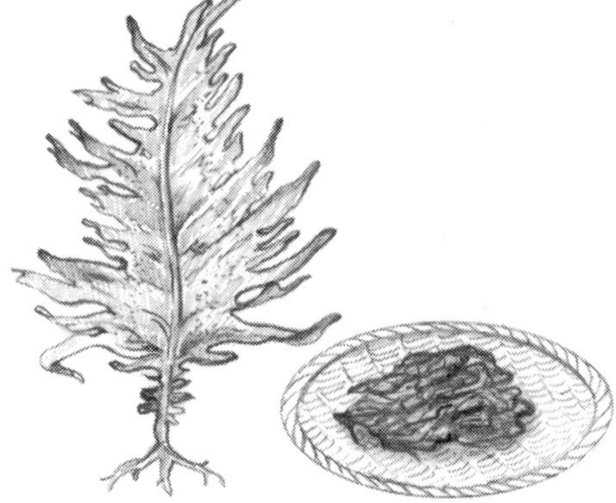

Fig. 21 Wakame

Wakame and Onions

1 oz. dried wakame
3 small onions, sliced
Tamari soy sauce, about 1–2 tsp.

Wash, soak, and slice the wakame into 1-inch pieces. Put the wakame and onions in a pot, side by side. Add enough soaking water to almost cover the sea vegetable. Bring to a boil, reduce heat to low, and simmer for 30 minutes, or until tender. Some varieties take longer to cook than others. Add tamari soy sauce to taste and cook for 10 to 15 minutes longer.

4. *Nori:* Nori comes in thin, flat, paper-like sheets. No washing, soaking, or cooking is required except to lightly toast it over an

open flame for a few seconds. In Japan it is used to garnish noodles, grains, and vegetables, and as a wrapping for sushi and rice balls, among other things.

Toast the nori by waving the dull side over the flame on an open gas burner. After toasting the sheets, they can be torn or cut with scissors, or left whole. Very small pieces or slivers make a good decorative garnish on top of noodles, grains, vegetables, and so on. One-eighth of a sheet is a nice size for covering and picking up small pieces of grains or vegetables. Two pieces (a quarter sheet) are used to wrap a rice ball.

Watercress Sushi

2 bunches watercress, washed, boiled 1 minute, drained
4 sheets nori, toasted
8–10 strips shiso leaves
2 Tbsps. toasted sesame seeds

Quickly rinse watercress under cold water to stop the cooking process. Then squeeze out excess liquid. Place a sheet of nori on a bamboo sushi mat. Cover about ¾ of the sheet of nori with a thin layer of watercress. Place 2 to 3 shiso leaves in a straight line across the watercress. Sprinkle some sesame seeds on top of the shiso.

Roll up as for regular sushi. Before unrolling the mat, squeeze gently to remove excess liquid. Quickly slice the roll into 6 to 8 equal-sized pieces or rounds. (If you do not roll and slice quickly, the nori falls apart.) Repeat until all ingredients are used up.

Norimaki (Sushi)
(See chapter on *Grains*.)

Rice Ball (Musubi)
(See chapter on *Grains*.)

5. *Dulse:* Dulse can be added raw or slightly toasted to soups, salads, and vegetable, grain, and bean dishes, at the very end of preparation, for extra flavor. It can also be lightly toasted by itself, crumbled and used as a condiment.

6. *Agar-agar:* Agar-agar is used as a jelling agent for kantens and aspics. It can be purchased in the form of bars or powder, and comes with cooking instructions enclosed. (See *Desserts* section for kanten recipes.)

13. Seasonings, Condiments, Sauces and Dressings

Besides ingredients and cooking methods, seasonings and condiments play a vital part in the balancing of a meal. As with any other aspect of preparing foods, care must be taken to have enough variety. The chart below lists some of the condiments mentioned in this book. They are categorized into the five tastes. Making sure to use items from each column insures a well-rounded diet.

SOUR	*BITTER*	*SWEET*	*PUNGENT*	*SALTY*
Pickles	Gomashio	Miso	Ginger	Miso
Sauerkraut	Tekka	Amazaké	Scallions	Gomashio
Umeboshi	Green nori	Applesauce	Onions	Umeboshi
Shiso leaves	Parsley	Rice syrup	Grated daikon	Shiso leaves
Rice vinegar	Dandelion	Barley malt	Watercress	Shio kombu
Lemon	Wakame powder	Mirin		Wakame powder
	Mustard greens (pickled)	Raisins		Tamari soy sauce
				Tekka

Seasonings:

1. *Sea salt:* Salt is one of the building blocks of life and we cannot survive without it. It is one of the basic ingredients of our blood and gives us vitality, strength, and mental clarity. Learning how to adjust salt intake and finding its balance with oil and water is an important part of mastering the art of cooking.

   Use only white unrefined sea salt. In commercial table salt, much of the valuable trace minerals have been removed. Sugar (dextrose), magnesium and sodium carbonate, and potassium iodine have been added in their place. Such salt depletes important minerals from the body and contributes to high blood pressure, heart problems, kidney disorders, and illness in general. Grey sea salt is also not recommended as it can cause excessive tightness in the body.

   The amount of salt that an individual needs depends on personal condition, age, activity level, and seasonal and other environmental factors. Physically active people, adults, persons with a more vegetarian-based history, and persons that live in a more wet, humid, and cold climate, can take more salt. (Babies should not take salt at all. It should be gradually introduced to their diet as they grow.) Individuals with a history of heavy meat consumption should carefully limit their salt intake and may even need to abstain for a short period of time. (These are the persons that benefit from vegetarian, raw food, and salt-free diets, which help to cleanse their bodies. However, after a while, salt and cooked foods should be reintroduced.)

Too much salt can cause hyperactivity, irritability, kidney problems, thirst and anger, among other things. Too little salt can cause poor circulation, mental lethargy, sleepiness, weakness, and so on. (Excess salt can also cause these symptoms at times.)

Meals should not be overwhelmingly salty. Salt should enhance and draw out the natural flavor and sweetness of foods, not cover them up. Generally, if, after meals, one becomes extremely thirsty or craves fatty, rich foods or strongly yin items such as sugar, ice cream, and so on, it is likely that an excess of salty (or hot) condiments and dishes have been consumed. Salt is very yang and attracts much yin, so too much makes it difficult to eat in a centered manner.

Plain salt is not recommended for use at the table. (An exception may be a small pinch on fresh fruits to draw out their sweetness.) It is too strong and difficult to assimilate in that form. Various condiments which substitute for salt—such as sea-vegetable powders or a mixture of salt and sesame seeds—are recommended. (See the *Condiments* section in this chapter.)

2. *Miso:* Miso is a paste made of fermented soybeans and sea salt which has been aged for a period of a few months to as much as three years or more. Miso only a few months old is light in color and contains less salt. If older, the color becomes a dark brown, and more salt is used to keep it going.

   The darker, longer-time miso is best for healing and is the kind that is assumed when using miso is recommended. The best miso is at least two summers old. There are three basic kinds now available in natural food stores. (Do not buy miso from Oriental food shops. It may be made without using a natural fermenting process, and also may contain chemicals and sugars.)

   A. *Hatcho miso:* Hatcho miso is 100 percent soybeans and is the darkest, most yang variety. It is especially recommended for the cold winter months.

B. *Mugi miso:* Mugi miso contains barley, is the sweetest of the three, and can be used all year round. It also has medicinal properties.

C. *Genmai (brown rice) or Kome (white rice) miso:* These misos contain rice. They are lighter and are good for the summer though they can also be used year round. Use this variety less often than the first two.

The short-term miso comes in red, yellow, or white. It is sweet, good for summer use, and makes delicious sauces and spreads but does not have medicinal value.

Buying bulk miso is recommended over the packaged variety, especially when one is trying to heal oneself, as it is more alive. Before being packaged, miso has to be pasteurized, otherwise it will keep fermenting and may burst its container.

Keep the bulk miso in a cool, dark place, and stir it from time to time. (The short-term kind should be refrigerated.) If a white color starts to appear on the surface, mix it into the bulk of the miso. This substance is a natural bacterial growth and is not harmful. On the contrary, besides adding more minerals and flavor to the miso, it is a reassurance that the miso is organic and alive.

3. *Tamari soy sauce and/or shoyu:* Tamari soy sauce is a liquid by-product of the miso-making process. It contains fermented soybeans, water, sea salt, and sometimes a small amount of wheat. Be very careful to avoid commercial shoyu as it is artificially aged and is full of chemicals and coloring. To be on the safe side, purchase soy sauce from natural food stores instead of Oriental ones.

   Tamari soy sauce can be added to just about any kind of dish for extra flavor. There are numerous recipes which use it throughout this book.

   Like salt and miso, tamari soy sauce should always be cooked into foods, not added afterward at the table, as this can cause tightness, produce cravings for sweets, and disrupt digestion. Also, be careful not to take too much of it.

4. *Umeboshi plum, paste, and vinegar, and shiso-leaf pickle:* Umeboshi plums have very strong medicinal value. They purify the bloodstream, detoxify poisons, stimulate appetite, and at times can help to relieve stomachaches, nausea, and air sickness. (Take them along whenever traveling.) When someone is not feeling well, we separate the meat of the plums from the pit, grind it into

a paste in a suribachi, or just chop it very finely, and add it to a thick kuzu drink (see *Special Needs* chapter), or serve it with rice cream.

Umeboshi plums have been pickled in sea salt and shiso leaves (to give the plums their bright red color) for a year or more. They can be added to just about any dish and may be used as a substitute for salt, tamari soy sauce, or miso. One plum is a delicious condiment with a bowl of rice or other grains. (See *Grains and Grain Products* chapter for a rice ball recipe.)

Recently, umeboshi paste and umeboshi vinegar (leftover juice from making these pickles) have become available. They are very handy to cook with and can be added to various dishes. However, they do not have the strong healing qualities of the plum. Therefore, when making *Special Needs* recipes or when trying to relieve a stomachache (for instance) use the whole plum.

Pickled shiso leaves are also available by themselves. They can be sliced and added to dishes in addition to, or as a substitute for, salt. They are valuable when dried or baked and ground into a powder for use as a condiment. In this form, they are helpful for neutralizing strong chemicals in the system.

5. *Oil:* Vegetable oils, which are full of polyunsaturated fatty acids, are needed to build new cells and tissues, to keep warm, for vitamins A and E, to maintain proper metabolism, and to lubricate skin and hair, among other things. However, much of the oil we need is already found in grains, beans, and seeds, so the intake of extra oil can be kept to a minimum, especially during the initial few months of healing. A healthy person can have a small amount of extra oil nearly every day in a side dish of sautéed vegetables or in a sauce or dressing. Even then, one or two tablespoons are adequate to sauté enough vegetables and grains for a whole family. Also, deep-fried foods should not be consumed more than once a week.

   Choose unrefined and cold-pressed oils (meaning that the seeds have been pressed below the boiling point and filtered). Such oils have all their vitamins and nutrients intact, are rich in color, retain the flavor and taste of the original seeds, and are somewhat cloudy in appearance. Please avoid refined oils or oils that have been processed at a high temperature.

   Animals oils and fats should be totally avoided as they contain high levels of cholesterol which causes hardening of the arteries and heart disease, among other things.

   To digest more oily foods such as fried rice, accompany them with grated ginger, or grated, raw daikon, or plenty of chopped raw scallions.

Keep oils in a tightly sealed container in a cool, dark place, or in the refrigerator.

Sesame oil, especially the dark variety made from roasted seeds, is the most healthy oil to use as it is easiest to digest and more yang than other varieties. Pumpkin seed oil is an occasional variation, and is also more yang than other oils.

Corn oil (a lighter oil for pastries or pie crusts), safflower, sunflower, and olive oil may all be used occasionally once sound health is established. It is best to avoid them until then.

6. *Brown Rice Vinegar:* Brown rice vinegar is to be used occasionally. It is delicious in sushi, dressings, grain salads, and pickles.

7. *Mirin:* Mirin is a cooking wine made from sweet rice. It is delicious in sweet-and-sour sauces, as well as in beans, vegetables, noodle broths, dressings, and marinades. Use this occasionally; it may be avoided initially for several months.

8. *Ginger:* Ginger is a hot, pungent, and very delicious root which stimulates the appetite, and activates circulation.

   A small amount of grated ginger spices up grains, vegetables, and noodles. Extract the juice by squeezing the grated ginger. (The juice is stronger.) Ginger is taken raw or added at the very end of preparations.

Fig. 22 Ginger

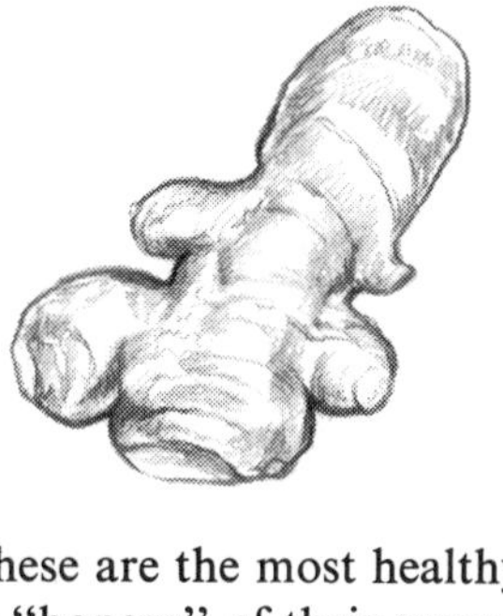

9. *Rice syrup and barley malt:* These are the most healthy sweeteners that we use. They are the "honeys" of their respective grains, and are delicious in desserts or cooked in with azuki or black soybeans.

Condiments:

Condiments, though we use them sparingly, are an indispensable part of macrobiotic eating. They add one or more of the following to a meal: color, extra variety and flavor, extra vitamins and minerals, appetite stimulation, balance, zest, and in some cases, medicinal value.

A small amount of various condiments may be used every day to accompany grains. They allow individuals to adjust their intake of salt, minerals, or oils to fit their personal needs. They are easy to overuse so be careful, especially when dealing with the saltier varieties such as gomashio or tekka.

Gomashio

(Gomashio, the most commonly used condiment in the Macrobiotic diet, is a perfect balance of salt and oil.)

14–16 Tbsps. black or white sesame seeds
1 level Tbsp. sea salt

Dry-roast sea salt in a skillet until it becomes shiny. (Roasting releases moisture in the salt and this helps to make a fluffier gomashio.) Place the roasted salt in a suribachi, and gently grind it to a fine powder.

Wash and rinse the sesame seeds and drain them in a fine wire-mesh strainer. Place them (they should still be wet) in a skillet and dry-roast them until they pop, emit a nutty fragrance, and can be crushed easily between the thumb and index fingers. Be careful not to burn them.

Place the seeds in the suribachi with the salt and grind them together until the seeds are half crushed and are all coated with salt. Make gentle circular motions using the grooves on the sides of the suribachi. When the gomashio cools, place it in an airtight glass or ceramic container. (If it is still warm, moisture will collect inside the container and can cause spoilage.) Sprinkle gomashio over grains and vegetables.

Sesame seeds are high in calcium, protein, iron, phosphorous, vitamin A, and niacin.

Scallion-Miso Condiment

2 bunches scallions
2 Tsps. miso
1 capful rice vinegar
Spring water

Separate scallion roots and greens. Blanch the roots 1 minute in a small amount of boiling water, and the greens for about 30 seconds. Dilute the miso with the rice vinegar and a small amount of boiling water. Simmer the miso mixture 2 to 3 minutes, cool slightly, and pour over the scallions, which have been placed on a serving dish.

Shio Kombu

8 long strips (about 12″) kombu
Enough liquid to cover (50% water and 50% tamari soy sauce)

Cut the kombu into 1-inch squares with scissors and soak them in water/tamari for 1 to 2 days. Place them into an uncovered pot, add enough water/tamari to cover, bring to a boil, immediately turn the flame to low, place a heat deflector underneath, and slowly simmer for several hours, until most of the liquid has evaporated. Since this is very strong, have only one or two pieces at a meal.

Nori Condiment

10 sheets nori, broken or cut into small pieces
1 cup spring water
½ Tbsp. tamari soy sauce

Bring all the ingredients to a boil in a small covered pot, turn the flame to low, and slowly simmer for about 20 to 30 minutes, or until most of the liquid has boiled away, leaving a paste of nori.

Wakame, Rice Vinegar Condiment

1 cup wakame, soaked and sliced
2 Tbsps. brown rice vinegar
2 Tbsps. soaking water from wakame
2 Tbsps. tamari soy sauce

Cook as in *Nori Condiment* (above), adding water, rice vinegar, and tamari soy sauce in the beginning with the wakame.

Wakame Powder

1 strip kombu, 10″

Gently wipe the wakame with a clean cloth to remove any surface sand or dust. Place it in a 350°F. oven for 10 to 15 minutes, or until it is crisp but not burnt. (While the wakame is in the oven, it may still seem wet. To test, remove a small piece and let it cool for a minute or two.) Grind the wakame to a fine powder in a suribachi. Use as a condiment for grains and vegetables.

Sauces and Dressings:

In general, it is best to use sauces and dressings sparingly. When properly prepared, most macrobiotic dishes are attractive and delicious enough to stand on their own. However, sauces and dressings can be a nice addition at times, particularly with more bland or lighter dishes, and for parties and special occasions. They can add appeal, like condiments, without covering up the taste and other qualities of the dish they accompany.

Kuzu Sauce

1–1½ cups soup or vegetable stock
1 Tbsp. kuzu dissolved in a small amount of water
Tamari soy sauce to taste
Optional: 2–3 pinches grated ginger

Bring dissolved kuzu and soup stock to a boil, lower the flame, and simmer and stir until the kuzu becomes transparent. Then add the tamari soy sauce and ginger. Serve over grains or vegetables.

Kuzu Sauce with Vegetables

½ carrot, cut into thin matchsticks
1 onion, thinly sliced
2 cups water or stock
2–2½ Tbsps. kuzu dissolved in a small amount of water
Tamari soy sauce to taste
***Optional:* a few pinches grated ginger, chopped scallions, or chopped parsley**

Bring the stock to a boil. Add the vegetables and simmer until almost soft. Add diluted kuzu and stir until the liquid becomes transparent. Add tamari soy sauce, simmer a few minutes more, and mix in scallions, parsley, or ginger if desired, just before serving.

Onion Butter

Enough thinly sliced onions to fill a pot
½" water
1–2 pinches sea salt

Fill a heavy-bottomed pot with onions. Add salt, about ½ inch of water, and cover the pot. Very slowly, on a low flame, bring this to a boil. Then, turn the flame down even lower, place a flame deflector under the pot, and simmer for 6 to 10 hours, until the onions dissolve to a golden brown paste.

Garnishes:

Garnishes are not to be forgotten in daily cooking. On one hand, they can delicately enhance the colors and appearance of your meals; on the other, they can add considerable dynamics in the areas of taste, texture, and energetics.

For instance, take a simple bowl of miso soup. By itself, it is strengthening and delicious. If you garnish that same bowl of soup (more yang) with fresh chopped scallions (more yin), the change is almost magical. The soup now is not only strengthening, but sweeter and more energizing as well.

Another example is a bowl of soba (buckwheat) noodles with tamari broth. Soba is a more yang food (tamari broth can be more yang also). A dish like this eaten without an added garnish, may leave you feeling heavy and weighted down. If you add fresh, grated ginger or chopped scallions (both much more yin than soba), the whole dish becomes much more charged. Not only are the colors more appealing, the sharp, pungent taste and the light, quick energy of scallions, (or the warm, active energy of ginger), make the soba a lot more zippy and energizing.

Some of the garnishes you could use are:

Chopped scallions
Chopped parsley
Chives
Chopped or grated onion
Grated ginger
A sprig of watercress
A celery leaf
Sliced or grated red radish
Sliced or grated daikon
Croutons
Toasted nori, cut into thin strips
Toasted white or black sesame seeds
Toasted pumpkin or sunflower seeds
Toasted almonds or walnuts
Sea vegetable powder
Sautéed vegetables
A lemon wedge
Raw vegetables or fruits cut into decorative shapes: a carrot flower, a cucumber fan, etc.

Examples for using garnishes include:

a. A rich, nishime-style dish with chopped parsley mixed in after cooking.
b. Thick, black soybean soup with a carrot flower, a dab of ginger, and a celery leaf in each bowlful.

c. A large serving platter of plain greens or pressed salad with toasted seeds sprinkled over.
d. A broiled fish fillet with a lemon wedge and a sprig of parsley.
e Strawberry kanten with a few almond slivers on top.
f. Feel free to create your own combinations.

Dressings:

Umeboshi Dressing

2 umeboshi plums
1/4–1/2 tsp. minced onion
1/2 tsp. sesame oil
1/2 cup spring water

Purée the umeboshi and onion in a suribachi. Heat the oil for about 1 minute and add it to the other ingredients. Add the water and mix well.

Sour Tofu Dressing

3 umeboshi plums
Spring water
1 cake tofu
1/4 cup sliced scallions or chives, for garnish

Put the pitted umeboshi plums in a suribachi and puree to a smooth paste. Add the tofu and puree until smooth and creamy, adding a little spring water to moisten, if necessary. Garnish with sliced scallions or chives. A little tamari soy sauce may be added to this recipe.

Miso-Rice Vinegar Dressing

2 tsps. miso
1/2 cup spring water
2 tsps. brown rice vinegar

Purée the miso in a little water in a suribachi then place in a pot and simmer for 2 to 3 minutes. Add the vinegar and the rest of the water and blend.

Tamari-Vinegar Dressing

***Optional:* 1/4–1/2 tsp. sesame oil**
1 Tbsp. tamari soy sauce
4 Tbsps. brown rice vinegar

1 Tbsp. fresh, grated onion
½ cup spring water

If using oil, heat it for about 1 minute over a low heat. Puree all the ingredients together in a suribachi and serve.

For variation:

1) **Miso and tamari are interchangeable.**
2) **Umeboshi is interchangeable with miso and tamari though it does not go well with rice vinegar or lemon.**
3) **Ginger, onions, parsley, scallions, and chives are interchangeable and can be used singularly or in combination. Using more than two at one time can get a bit too complicated.**
4) **Lemon can be substituted for rice vinegar.**

14. Desserts

Delicious desserts can be made using squash, sweet grains, or azuki beans as a base, rather than fruit or flour. The best sweeteners for health are:

1. Amazaké, a drink or a pudding made from fermented sweet rice and a starter called koji, also made from rice. It can be consumed as it is, or added to other dessert recipes.
2. Rice syrup
3. Barley malt syrup
4. Chestnuts
5. Mirin, a cooking wine made from sweet rice. It is used more in regular cooking than in desserts
6. Raisins and other dried fruits such as apples, peaches, pears, apricots, currants, and cherries
7. Fresh seasonal fruits, cooked
8. Apple juice and cider

Agar-agar and kuzu are natural thickeners which can be used in place of eggs, gelatin, and the like.

For more extensive recipes on cookies, cakes, muffins, and so on, refer to other macrobiotic cookbooks. Since this book deals mainly with the healing process, these less healthful types of desserts are not included.

Amazaké
(Also sold ready-made in some natural food stores.)

4 cups sweet brown rice
½ cup koji (sold in some natural food stores)
8 cups water

Soak the rice overnight and pressure-cook it for 30 minutes. When done, place it into a glass bowl and, as soon as it becomes cool enough to handle, mix in the koji, cover with a towel, and put it in a warm place. An oven with just the pilot light on, or the radiator, will do. Let this ferment for 4 to 8 hours. Mix it once in a while to help dissolve the koji. The fermentation is done when bubbles start to appear on the surface and when the mixture begins to taste sweet. It becomes sweeter and sweeter up to a certain point and then starts to turn sour. Catch it when it is sweet, place it back into a pot, bring it to a boil, add a pinch of salt, and turn it off as soon as it starts to bubble.

Amazaké can be used as it is or blended in a food mill. For a delicious drink, after blending, add a small amount of water and optional grated ginger, bring to a boil, and serve. Or, let it cool off to make a refreshing cold beverage.

To keep the amazaké for a longer time, simmer it over a low flame with a heat deflector underneath until it becomes slightly brown.

Basic Amazaké Pudding

4 cups amazake drink
6 Tbsps. kuzu, dissolved in a small amount of water
2 pinches sea salt
***Optional:* 1/4 cup raisins**

Place all ingredients into a pot, and bring to a boil while stirring constantly with a wooden spoon to avoid lumping and burning. Then simmer for about 3 minutes, pour into a serving plate, let it set, garnish, and serve. If it jelled properly, you will be able to slice it into squares. Serves 8.

Corn Amazake

Amazake can be made from corn but it is a little more complicated to make than the brown rice variety. First cook the corn as in the *Arepa* recipe (see chapter 8 on *Grains*). Grind the cooked corn, then mix it together with koji starter. From this point, prepare in the same way as for rice amazake.

Chestnut Sweet Rice

2 cups sweet rice
1/2 cup dried chestnuts
3 cups spring water
2 pinches sea salt

Wash the chestnuts (sort out the discolored ones) and dry-roast them for about 5 minutes in a skillet over a medium-low flame. Stir with a wooden spoon, making sure that they do not burn. Put them in a pressure cooker with sweet rice and cook as in *Basic Brown Rice*. Serves 4 to 6.

Sweet Azuki Beans

1 cup azuki beans
1 cup chestnuts
⅛ cup raisins (or ½ cup rice syrup)
5 cups water
½ tsp. sea salt

Soak azuki beans and chestnuts for 6 to 8 hours or overnight. Place all the ingredients except salt into a pressure cooker and pressure-cook for 40 to 45 minutes. Let the pressure come down completely. Add salt, bring to a boil again, turn flame to low, and simmer for another 15 to 20 minutes. Or, you can simmer for a longer time, in which case it will become even sweeter.

Ohagi

(See recipe in Chapter 8.)

Rice Pudding

4 cups cooked brown rice
3 cups apple cider
½ cup raisins, soaked
Rind of ½ lemon, finely chopped
1 pinch sea salt

Place all ingredients in a pot and bring to a boil. Reduce heat and simmer 30 to 45 minutes. Garnish with roasted, chopped almonds, or apple chunks cooked with a little water, rice syrup, and grated ginger.

Squash Pudding

1 medium-sized buttercup squash (about 2½–3 lbs.)
1 cup spring water
1 pinch sea salt
¼–½ cup barley malt
1 Tbsp. kuzu
1 cup chopped walnuts

Wash squash and remove skin and seeds. Cut squash into chunks and place in a pot with the water. Add a pinch of sea salt, bring to a boil, reduce heat to medium-low, and cover. Simmer until the squash is soft, about 20 minutes. Puree the squash in a hand food mill until smooth.

Return the pureed squash to the pot and add the barley malt.

Simmer for about 5 minutes. Dilute the kuzu in a little water and add it to the pureed squash, stirring constantly to avoid lumping. Simmer for 2 to 3 minutes. Remove from the heat and allow to cool slightly. Pour into serving dishes. Serves 4 to 6.

Couscous Cake

2 pints amazake
2 pints apple juice
2 pints spring water
4 cups couscous (dry)
1 pinch sea salt
Grated rind of two lemons

Combine all liquid ingredients in a saucepan and bring to a boil. Add couscous, salt, and lemon rind, and simmer 15 minutes. Put in an 8-inch cake pan which has been rinsed in cold water. Bake at 350°F. approximately 15 minutes, or until the cake begins to come away from the edges of the pan. Cool and top with apple butter, unsweetened preserves, or fruit glazed with kuzu.

Sweet Kuzu

1 tsp. kuzu
1 Tbsp. rice syrup or barley malt syrup
1 cup water

Dissolve the kuzu in 2 teaspoons of cold water until it becomes a liquid. Put this in a pot with remaining water and sweetener. Stirring constantly with a wooden spoon, bring this mixture to a boil, turn the flame to low, and simmer for 10 to 15 minutes. Serve hot.

Rice Syrup-Sesame Seed Kanten

2 cups water
2 cups rice syrup
½ cup sesame seeds
⅓ tsp. sea salt
1 bar agar-agar or 6 Tbsps. agar-agar flakes

Wash, dry-roast, and crush the sesame seeds into a fine powder in a suribachi. Then stir and boil all the ingredients and simmer for 15 minutes. Wet a mold and pour all the ingredients into it. Refrigerate for an hour or so until it jells. Serves 8.

Strawberry Kanten

2 cups strawberries
4 cups apple juice (or 2 cups juice and 2 cups water)
⅛ tsp. sea salt
1 bar agar-agar or 6 Tbsps. agar-agar flakes
1 Tbsp. kuzu diluted in a little cold water

Bring the liquid, salt, agar-agar, and kuzu to a boil, turn the flame to low, simmer and keep stirring until the kuzu becomes transparent and the agar-agar dissolves completely. Add the strawberries. Pour into a serving dish or bowl which has been rinsed with cold water. This dish can be varied by using other dried or fresh fruits and/or nuts. Serves 8.

Azuki Kanten

1 cup azuki beans
1½ cups raisins
4 cups spring water
5 Tbsps. agar-agar flakes
3 cups spring water
1 piece kombu, 3″

Soak azuki beans 6 to 8 hours and cook with raisins, kombu, and 4 cups water in a pressure-cooker for 1 hour. Dissolve agar-agar in remaining 3 cups water, add to the beans, and cook for another 5 minutes. Cool and pour into a serving dish or bowl. This dish can be made with apple juice instead of water, or the water may be sweetened with barley malt.

Applesauce

8 apples, cored
Water
2 pinches sea salt
***Optional:* 1 Tbsp. kuzu (For those with an overly yin condition.)**

Cut apple into 1½-inch slices and place in a pot. Add about 1 inch of water and the sea salt. Bring to a boil, and simmer over low heat until apples are soft. Puree in a food mill and serve.

Peach Pie

8 ripe peaches
⅛ tsp. sea salt
½ cup kuzu

Cut peaches in half and remove pits. Slice into 1-inch pieces.

Grind kuzu and salt to a fine powder in a suribachi. Mix with peaches.

4 cups whole wheat pastry flour
½ cup corn oil
2 Tbsps. barley malt
2 pinches sea salt
Cold water

Mix together the flour and salt. Add oil and quickly and gently mix until it forms small beads in the flour. Add barley malt and enough water to form a dough, mixing quickly and gently. (Do not over-mix, as it will make the crust tough. The less the better.)

Separate the dough into two balls, one slightly larger than the other (this is for the bottom crust). Dust a sheet of wax paper with flour and place the dough on it. Cover with another layer of waxed paper and roll out the larger piece of dough between the two sheets (quickly and gently).

When the dough is about ¼-inch thick, transfer it to a pie plate. Add peach filling and roll out the other piece of dough. Lay it on top of the pie, trimming and sealing the edges where the two crusts meet. Cut a few holes on the top crust to let steam escape while baking.

Bake at 350°F. for 45 minutes. Turn heat to 425°F. and cook for 15 minutes more. Wait until cool before slicing. (You can put a cookie sheet on the rack under the pie while it is cooking to catch any drippings.)

Mochi Pie Crust

(This is a much healthier alternative to regular pie crust but is only practical for open-faced pies.)
Cook and pound sweet rice as in the *Mochi* recipe, but then, instead of using it as mochi, oil a pie plate and press the mochi into it and shape it as a pie crust. Then bake as usual. This does not need to be prebaked before adding filling.

This crust makes the most delicious vegetable pies. Tofu, seitan, tempeh, or natto can also be added. (For vegetable pies, a small condiment of grated daikon with tamari soy sauce or grated ginger will make a nice complement. This is not necessary for sweetened or fruit pies.)

Squash Pie

1 large cubed and peeled buttercup squash

1 cup barley malt
¼ tsp. sea salt
¼ cup water
½ cup dry-roasted, chopped walnuts

Pressure-cook squash, barley malt, water, and salt. Puree in a food mill. Place in a pot and simmer for 10 minutes. If it is too thick, add some more water. If it is too thin, cook until it thickens. It should be pretty thick. (Kuzu can also be added to thicken it.) Place in a prebaked pie shell and sprinkle chopped walnuts on top. Bake at 350° to 365°F. for ½ hour, or until the crust is golden brown.

For a crust, use a mochi crust or half of the pie crust recipe from the *Peach Pie* recipe. (Bake crust at 425°F. for 10 to 15 minutes, or until golden brown.)

Chestnuts, fresh fruits, and other vegetables (unsweetened) can also be used as filling. Try making an onion pie with sautéed onions.

Dried Apricot Purée Topping

1 cup unsulfured dried apricots
2 cups water
Pinch of sea salt
2 Tbsps. kuzu, diluted

Pressure-cook apricots in sea salt and water for 25 to 30 minutes. Bring pressure down. Purée apricots and liquid in a hand food mill. Place this mixture back in the pressure cooker. Add diluted kuzu, stirring constantly until thick. Eat as is or use as a topping for couscous cake. Serves 4.

Dried Fruit Compote

¼ cup raisins or currants
½ cup dried apples
½ cup dried apricots
3 cups spring water
2 Tbsps. kuzu

Soak raisins or currants, apples, and apricots in water at least 30 minutes. Add a pinch of sea salt to the fruit and bring to a boil over medium heat. Cover and simmer 20 minutes. Dilute kuzu with a little cold water. Reduce heat to low and add the kuzu to the fruit. Stir constantly until thick, simmer for 2 to 3 minutes, and serve.

15. Fish

Fish should be eaten as fresh as possible, preferably the same day it is caught, or at least the same day it is purchased. Choose more yin, slow-moving, soft white-meat fish such as sole, flounder, haddock, carp, and so on, as opposed to more active, red-meat varieties such as tuna, salmon, swordfish, and the like. Temporarily avoid shellfish such as clams, oysters, mussels, shrimp, lobster, and crab.

It may be best for some persons to avoid fish entirely, at least for several months, or until symptoms have improved.

Eat two or three times the regular amount of hard leafy greens when including fish in a meal to help balance its strong yang energies. Grated daikon with a few drops of tamari and a bit of grated ginger will help neutralize any possible toxic side-effects of the fish. A few drops of lemon is helpful and a slice of lemon is a beautiful garnish as well.

Clear Fish Soup

1–2 fillets of sole (or other white-meat fish)
1 cup wakame, soaked and cut into 1″ slices
1 bunch watercress, previously boiled for 1 second
3 shiitake mushrooms, soaked and sliced
5–6 cups kombu stock (add shiitake soaking water)
Tamari soy sauce to taste

Bring wakame, shiitake, and kombu stock to a boil, turn the flame down, and simmer for a few minutes until the wakame and shiitake soften. Cut the fish into 1½- to 2-inch pieces, and add them to the soup with tamari to taste. Simmer for 1 to 2 minutes or until the fish turns white. Ladle the soup into individual serving bowls and garnish with the watercress. Serves 6 to 8.

Fish Stew

1 lb. cod (or other white-meat fish)
½ cup onions, chunks
½ cup carrot, chunks
¼ cup celery, sliced on thick diagonal
½ cup daikon, chunks
2 Tbsps. burdock, shaved
1 strip kombu, 6″–8″, soaked and cubed

6 cups water
Tamari soy sauce to taste
Scallion garnish

Place kombu, vegetables, and water in a pot. Bring to a boil, cover, reduce flame, and simmer several minutes, until the vegetables are tender. Cut fish into 2-inch chunks and place them in the pot with vegetables. Simmer 5 to 7 minutes. Add tamari soy sauce to taste and simmer another 2 to 3 minutes. Garnish and serve. Serves 5 to 6.
Occasionally, for a thicker stew, add 4 to 5 teaspoons of diluted kuzu to thicken the stew at end of cooking

Koi Koku (Carp Soup)

1 small carp (about 2 lbs.)
Equal volume of thinly shaved burdock and/or carrots
1 cup bancha tea twigs and leaves (already used to make tea)
Enough liquid to cover, ⅓ bancha and ⅔ water
Grated ginger
Miso to taste, puréed
Clean 100% cotton cheesecloth

Buy a fresh carp, preferably a live one and ask the fish seller to kill and carefully remove the gallbladder and the yellow bitter thyroid bone. Leave the rest of the fish intact.

At home, chop the whole fish (bones, head, fins included) into 1-inch pieces.

Make a sack out of the cheesecloth and put the used bancha tea twigs inside. This helps to soften the fish bones.

Place all the ingredients, including the sack of tea twigs, but not the miso, into a pressure cooker. Pressure-cook for 1½ to 2 hours. Bring down the pressure, take off the lid, add the ginger and miso to taste, simmer for 5 minutes, and serve. Garnish with chopped scallions. Serves 6 to 8.

Baked Scrod with Miso

1 cup barley miso
1 cup white miso
2 Tbsps. saké
½ cup mirin
1½–2 lbs. scrod fillets
Grated daikon

Puree the miso, mirin, and saké together thoroughly in a suribachi. Spread half the marinade over the bottom of a shallow baking dish. Lay the fish fillets on top of the miso spread. Then spread the remaining marinade on top. Let sit for 4 to 5 hours. Remove the fish from the marinade. Put the marinated fish in a baking dish and bake in a preheated 475°F. oven for 15 to 20 minutes. Serve with grated daikon.

Broiled Marinated Haddock

1½ lbs. fresh haddock fillets
3 Tbsps. tamari soy sauce
2 Tbsps. mirin
Lemon wedges

Rinse fish and pat dry. Combine the tamari soy sauce and mirin in a baking dish, and place the fish in the marinade, turning to coat both sides. Let the fish remain in the marinade about 15 minutes per side, basting occasionally.

Preheat the broiler. Place the fish fillets on a lightly oiled baking sheet, and pour a little marinade over them. Broil the fish 3 to 5 minutes, turn, spoon on a little more marinade, and broil another 3 minutes, or until the fish is thoroughly cooked. Remove fish to a serving plate and garnish with lemon wedges.

16. Beverages

It is best to drink only when thirsty. Most of us drink out of habit, whether we want to or not (as we often do with eating). If often or strongly thirsty, some of the dietary reasons may include:

1) **Overconsumption of salt**
2) **Overconsumption of animal products**
3) **Overconsumption of dry, baked and/or flour products**
4) **Overconsumption of spices**
5) **Overconsumption of food in general**
6) **Not chewing enough**
7) **Lack of fresh, light dishes**
8) **Excess of sea vegetables**

Good-quality water, such as spring or well water is the best to use. Avoid distilled or highly chemicalized tap water as much as possible.

It is also best to avoid iced or cold drinks (even water), as they can shock and paralyze the digestive system and harden fat accumulations in the body.

The beverages used on a daily basis do not contain caffeine, sugar, carbonation, artificial color, preservatives, stimulants, or alcohol (particularly the hard-liquor varieties). If following the general "standard diet," occasional small quantities of more yin, good-quality drinks, such as green tea, beer, saké, and mint teas can be consumed. However, if an individual is trying to reverse a particular condition, these items are best avoided.

The recipes in the *Special Needs* chapter are to be used only when really necessary, and only for a short period of time.

Bancha Twig Tea (Kukicha)
(For daily use, the "brown rice" of beverages.)

1–2 Tbsps. bancha twigs
1½ quarts of water

Twig tea generally comes pre-roasted. If not, dry-roast the whole package of twigs and leaves in a skillet for 3 to 4 minutes, stirring gently with a wooden spoon. Set aside the 1 to 2 tablespoons to be used, and store the rest, after cooling, in an airtight jar until needed.

Add twigs to cold water, bring them to a boil, reduce the

flame to low, and simmer 10 to 15 minutes, depending on the strength desired. While pouring tea into individual cups, use a bamboo tea strainer (available in natural or Oriental food stores) to strain out the twigs. A regular metal strainer can be used as an alternative. The twigs may be reused several times until they lose their strength, but make fresh tea on a regular basis.

Kukicha contains no caffeine, artificial colorings, or dyes, and is not aromatic. It aids digestion and helps to settle an acidic stomach as it is alkaline in nature. (Most teas are acidic.)

Kukicha or bancha is made from the twigs and leaves of an older, matured tea bush, named *ban* in Japanese. (*Cha* is the Japanese word for tea. Hence, saying "bancha tea" is really saying *ban* tea tea.)

The same bush also supplies some green tea which is made from the topmost and youngest, greenest leaves. This tea is delicious but contains much caffeine and is not recommended for regular use. As the bush becomes older, the caffeine content begins to decrease and finally disappears. Harvesting different sections of the plant, and at different stages in its growth, produces a variety of teas.

Homemade Grain Teas
(Good for daily or regular use.)

To make grain tea, wash and dry-roast any grain, including rice, millet, oats, barley, and wheat, in a dry skillet. Use a wooden spoon to stir. Store what is not needed immediately in an airtight container, after cooling, for later use. Take 2 tablespoons for 1½ to 2 quarts of water and boil and simmer as in bancha tea.

Mugicha (Roasted Unhulled Barley Tea)
(Good for daily or regular use.)

2 Tbsps. mugicha (available in natural food stores)
1½–2 quarts of water

Place the mugicha in cold water, bring it to a boil, reduce the flame to low, and simmer several minutes. Cooking time depends on the strength of tea desired.

Yannoh/Grain Coffee/Root Coffee
(For more "occasional use.")

4 tsp. yannoh
4 cups of water

Bring yannoh and 4 cups of cold water to a boil. Immediately reduce the flame (as it will boil over), and simmer for several minutes.

Yannoh is sold in natural food stores but may be difficult to find. (When buying grain coffee, make sure that it does not contain fruits or more yin vegetables such as beets.) Below is a recipe for homemade yannoh.

Yannoh (Homemade)

3 cups brown rice
2½ cups wheat berries
1½ cups azuki beans
2 cups chick-peas
1 cup chicory root

Wash each ingredient, then separately dry-roast each until a nutty fragrance is emitted. Then grind and mix.

When cool, store the Yannoh in an airtight jar. For variety, experiment with different proportions of grains, beans, vegetables (like burdock or dandelion root), and chicory. One hundred percent dandelion-root coffee can be delicious.

Azuki Bean Tea
(For occasional use, and as a medicinal drink.)

1 cup azuki beans
3–4 cups water
1 piece kombu

Place kombu in the bottom of a pan, then add azuki beans and water. Boil, reduce flame to low, and simmer until the water becomes a rich red. Azuki tea is helpful when the kidneys are tight. Have one cup a day for 3 days.

Kombu Tea
(For "occasional use.")

1 strip kombu, 6″
2 cups water

Boil the kombu and water until only 1 cup of liquid remains.

Mu Tea
(For "occasional use" only.)

1 teabag Mu tea (sold in natural food stores)
4 cups water

Boil, reduce flame, and simmer for 10 minutes. Mu tea is made of a combination of either 9 or 16 different herbs. The mixture was concocted by my teacher, George Ohsawa, the man who first introduced macrobiotic principles to the Western countries.

Umeboshi Tea
(For "occasional use.")

3–4 umeboshi plums
1½–2 quarts water
Optional: 1–2 shiso leaves

Separate the meat of the umeboshi from the pits and tear it into several pieces. Add the umeboshi meat and pits to the water and bring to a boil. Turn the flame to low and simmer for 20 to 30 minutes. When cooled, this is a delicious, refreshing summer drink. It helps reduce thirst and replaces minerals lost by excessive sweating.

Leftover Vegetable Juice
(For "occasional use.")

The leftover liquid from boiling or pressure-cooking vegetables makes a nice beverage. Just make sure that there is not a lot of concentrated salt in the water.

Vegetable and Fruit Juices
(For "occasional use.")

The juice of any "regular use" vegetable or seasonal fruit on the *Standard Dietary Suggestions* list may be taken once in a while. In the winter it is preferable to heat juice up, especially the yinner fruit juices.

Carrot Juice

Place carrots in a juicer and grind. This is helpful for some forms of arthritis.

Dandelion Tea

2 Tbsps. chopped dandelion root
1 qt. spring water

Bring to a boil. Reduce flame to low, and simmer 7 to 10 minutes.

Sweet Vegetable Broth

1/4 cup chopped onion
1/4 cup chopped carrots
1/4 cup chopped cabbage
1/4 cup chopped green winter squash (buttercup or butternut)
3–4 cups spring water

Place vegetables and water in a pot, bring to a boil, and simmer about 15 to 20 minutes, or until the vegetables soften and release their sweetness into the liquid. Drink one to two cups per day. The cooked vegetables can also be eaten.

17. Special Needs

There are a variety of natural home remedies which may be helpful during the recovery process. For information about the duration of their use and the specific conditions for which they are recommended, please review the section in this book on *Dietary Adjustments for the Five Major Types of Arthritis*. Readers may also consult the companion book in the *Macrobiotic Health Education Series* as well as *Macrobiotic Home Remedies*, both by Michio Kushi.

Internal Remedies:

Agar-agar with Rice Syrup or Barley Malt
(To relieve constipation.)

1½ Tbsps. agar-agar flakes
1 Tbsp. rice syrup or barley malt
1 cup spring water
1 pinch sea salt

Bring all the ingredients to a boil, turn the flame down, and simmer 5 to 10 minutes. Remove the pot from the stove and take this drink while it is still warm.

Daikon Tea

2 Tbsps. grated daikon
A few drops tamari soy sauce
1 teacup hot bancha tea

Place daikon and tamari soy sauce in a drinking cup, fill the cup with hot bancha tea, stir, and drink. This drink may be used once a day for 2 to 3 days.

Carrot-Daikon Tea

1 Tbsp. grated carrot
1 Tbsp. grated daikon
A few drops tamari soy sauce
1 teacup hot bancha tea

Place the grated carrot and daikon, and the tamari soy sauce in a drinking cup, fill the cup with hot bancha tea, stir, and drink. This drink may be taken once a day for three days.

Kombu Tea

2 cups spring water
1 piece kombu, 3″–6″

Bring kombu and water to a boil, reduce the flame to low, and simmer until only 1 cup of water remains. Drink this two to three times per week.

Tamari Bancha

A few drops tamari soy sauce
1 teacup hot bancha tea

Place of few drops of tamari soy sauce into a teacup. Pour in hot bancha tea, stir, and drink. Use this drink on occasion, as needed.

Ume-Sho-Kuzu

1 heaping tsp. kuzu
1 tsp. tamari soy sauce
1 umeboshi plum, seed removed
1/8 tsp. fresh, grated ginger
1 cup spring water

Chop the meat of the umeboshi plum and put it aside. Dissolve the kuzu in a teaspoon of water until it becomes a liquid, then add it to a small pot with 1 cup of water. Bring this to a boil, then turn the flame to low, and stir constantly with a wooden spoon. When the mixture becomes transparent, add the tamari soy sauce, umeboshi, and ginger. Drink hot.

Shredded Daikon Tea

1/4 cup shredded, dried daikon
2 cups water
1 pinch sea salt

Boil the shredded, dried daikon (available in many natural food stores) in 2 cups of water and the sea salt until only 1 cup remains. Drink hot.

Lotus Seeds and Kombu

1/2 cup lotus seeds soaked overnight
1 strip kombu, 3″ soaked and cut into thin matchsticks
Tamari soy sauce
Enough water to cover seeds

Bring the lotus seeds, kombu, and water to a boil, then turn the flame to low and simmer about 30 minutes, until the seeds and kombu become soft. Then add a few drops of tamari soy sauce to taste and simmer another 5 minutes. You can also use fresh or dried lotus root.

External Treatments:

Ginger Compress

(Helps circulation, and softens and dissolves mucus, cysts, tumors, and the like.)

6 Tbsps. grated ginger
1 gallon water
Cheesecloth 6″ by 6″
Rubber gloves
3 cotton towels
Optional: hot plate
(A person to give the treatment. It is awkward and not relaxing to do it on oneself.)

Bring a pot of water to a boil and turn the flame off. Meanwhile, make a sack out of cheesecloth, place the grated ginger inside, and tie the open end into a knot to close it. Immediately after turning off the flame and the bubbles have disappeared, squeeze as much ginger liquid as possible out of the sack and into the pot of water. Then, place the whole bag inside. The point is to put the ginger in water as hot as possible without boiling it, as boiling would cancel its effectiveness.

Lay the person who will receive the ginger compress on a bed or some cushions and let him or her relax. Put on the rubber gloves. Holding on to the two ends of a cotton towel, dip as much of it as possible into the water. Wring it out, and place it on the area of the body to be treated. If it is too hot, shake the towel a bit before applying it. Ideally, the towel should be as hot as one can stand. Cover it with a dry cotton towel to keep it warm for a longer time. Place another towel in the water and when the first towel has cooled off, wring this one out and exchange it with the first. Again, cover with the dry towel. Continue alternating the towels until the area being treated becomes red. The water can be reheated (but not boiled) if it becomes too cool.

The ginger compress is a wonderfully effective home remedy. In addition, it is inexpensive, easy to apply, and has no harmful side effects. However, there are situations in which the ginger compress should be used only as a preliminary to another application, and there are situations where it should not be used at all. Please consult a qualified macrobiotic teacher for guidance. Also, the book, *Macrobiotic Home Remedies* (see bibliography), offers a thorough explanation of this and many other natural applications.

Buckwheat Plaster
(Draws out excess fluid from swollen areas.)

Buckwheat flour
Enough hot water to form a hard, stiff dough
5%–10% grated ginger
Clean cotton linen

Precede the plaster with a 5-minute application of the ginger compress on the swollen area. Form a dough with the flour, hot water, and ginger, and place a ½-inch layer on the affected area. Cover and tie it on with a strip of linen. Replace the buckwheat every 4 hours. The swelling should go down after several applications or at the most after 2 to 3 days.

Lotus Root Plaster
(Draws out excess mucus, especially from the sinuses, lungs, and bronchi.)

75%–85% grated fresh lotus root
10%–15% pastry flour
5%–10% grated ginger
Cotton linen

Mix these ingredients and spread them ½-inch thick onto a linen cloth. Apply the plaster directly to the skin on the area you are treating. Tie and keep this on for a few hours or

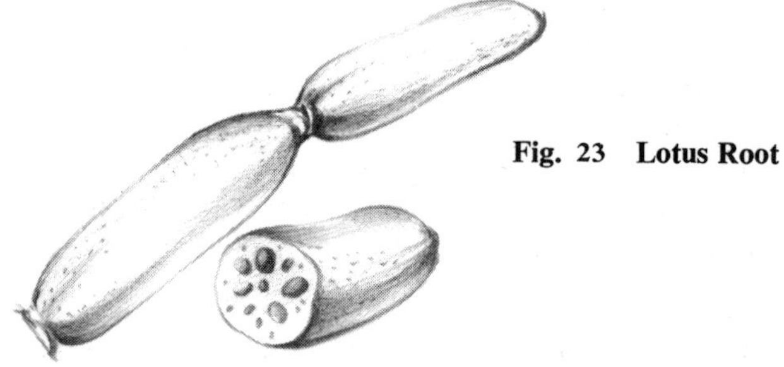

Fig. 23 Lotus Root

overnight, and repeat this for a few days. It is helpful to do a ginger compress on the area before applying the plaster.

Daikon-Leaf Hip Bath

(For female sexual organ troubles.)

4–5 bunches dried daikon leaves (if unavailable, substitute 2 handfuls sea salt or 1 cup dried arame sea vegetable)
4–5 quarts water
1 handful sea salt
A bathtub of waist-level hot water
A towel

Dry several bunches of fresh daikon or turnip greens in the shade, until they become dry and brittle. (Dried daikon leaves can also be purchased in some natural food stores.)

Boil the dried tops with the handful of salt until the 4 to 5 quarts of water turns brown. Straining out the leaves, pour the liquid into the bathtub. The water in the tub should be hot and should come up to waist level. With a towel covering the upper part of the body, sit in the tub until the whole body becomes warm and begins to sweat (about 10 minutes). Do this for as many days as needed. Follow the bath with a bancha tea douche (see below).

Bancha Tea Douche

(For female sexual organ troubles.)

Enough lukewarm bancha tea for douching
½ tsp. sea salt
Juice from half a lemon or equivalent amount of brown rice vinegar

Combine all the ingredients and use as a douche after taking the daikon leaf hip bath.

Greens with Bran Plaster

(Help to reduce discomfort from skin irritation or inflammation.)

50% rice bran
50% finely chopped, raw, green leafy vegetables
A little water to help make a paste
Cotton linen

Crush the hard, leafy, chopped greens (such as collards, kale, watercress, etc.) in a suribachi until they turn into a pulp. Combine with the bran and some water to make a paste. Apply the plaster on the feverish area and remove it when the paste becomes warm or hot.

Greens with Nori Plaster
(Helps to reduce discomfort from skin irritation or inflammation.)

Finely chopped raw, green leafy vegetables
A few sheets of nori

Crush the greens (such as collards, kale, watercress, etc.) and nori in a suribachi until they become a pulp. Apply this on the feverish area until the paste becomes warm or hot.

Tofu Plaster

1 cake fresh tofu
Equivalent amount of finely diced cabbage
Enough whole wheat flour to hold it together, about 10%–20% of the plaster.
1 tsp. grated ginger

Grind the tofu and cabbage into a paste in a suribachi. Add the ginger and flour, and place this mixture on a cheesecloth or cotton cloth, forming a sack with the tofu mixture inside. Put this on the forehead or any affected area, using the cheesecloth to tie it in place. When the mixture becomes warm, perhaps in 2 to 3 hours, exchange it for a fresh application.

Rice Bran Wash

Use two handfuls of rice bran (nuka). Make a sack out of a cotton cloth or cheesecloth (several layers thick), put in the bran and tie it tightly. Use this to scrub your body when you take a bath or shower. It can be used several times until it starts to spoil. This is also good for skin rashes.

Glossary

Agar-agar—A white gelatin made from sea vegetable, used for making *kanten*. You can get it in bars or flakes.

Ame—A natural grain honey derived from rice, barley, or wheat.

Amazake—A sweet porridge or drink made from fermented sweet rice. You can make this at home or buy it in some natural food stores.

Arame—A variety of sea vegetable.

Arepas—Corn cake made from *masa* corn dough.

Arrowroot—A finely ground white flour, used as a thickener, similar to *kuzu* and corn starch.

Azuki beans—Small, red beans. They are good for the kidneys.

Bancha—Tea made from a tea bush which is at least three years old. It helps digestion, and is good for daily use.

Burdock—A long, thin, dark, black root which grows all over the United States, as well as in other parts of the world. It gives one strength and stamina.

Couscous—A partially refined cracked wheat. It is light and cooks quickly. It is good for summer cooking.

Daikon—A long, thick, white root from the radish family. It is pungent when raw and is sweet when cooked. It is an excellent cleanser and purifier of blood, as it helps to break down fat deposits. Grated raw and served with a drop of *tamari* soy sauce, it is a good garnish with oily, greasy foods, making them more digestible.

Dulse—A variety of sea vegetable harvested in Maine, among other places.

Fu—Derived from wheat gluten, you can buy it in natural food stores in either flat, thin sheets, or in round donut shapes. When dry it is like a cracker but when cooked it is more like a noodle. A fun food.

Ginger—A hot, pungent, gnarly-looking, flesh-colored root. It adds zest to your dishes, and also helps circulation whether taken internally or applied externally as in a ginger compress.

Ginger compress—An external treatment made from grated ginger and hot water. It stimulates circulation, and unblocks stagnation (*see recipe*).

Gomashio—A condiment made from roasted sesame seeds and sea salt.

Hijiki—A black stringy variety of sea vegetable.

Hokkaido squash—A delicious squash, similar to buttercup.

Jinenjo—A very hardy, long, flesh-colored, mountain root potato. When grated it becomes a sticky mass and can be eaten with grains, or you can slice it and add it to vegetable dishes. It gives one strength.

Kanten—A gelatin-type food made from agar-agar. It makes a great light dessert when made with fruit and fruit juice. It is also used for aspics.

Kasha—Buckwheat groats.

Kinpira—A thinly sliced or shaved, sautéed-burdock dish, with or without carrots, and seasoned with *tamari* soy sauce.

Koji—Rice which has been innoculated with a form of bacteria. It is used as a starter for making *amazake*, *saké*, *miso*, and *tamari* soy sauce.

Kombu—A long, smooth, flat, thick variety of sea vegetable used in soup stocks, vegetable, bean, and grain dishes, and condiments.

Kukicha—Another name for *bancha*.

Kuzu—A starch made from the root of the *kuzu* plant (called *kudzu* in the United States), which is used as a thickener in vegetables dishes, and for medicinal purposes. When you buy it, it looks like little white rocks.

Lotus root—A tubular, flesh-colored root from the water lily family. It is hollowed out by several lengthwise airholes. It is good for the respiratory system and helps to unclog the sinuses.

Lotus seeds—Seeds of the above. They look like chick-peas.

Masa—A whole corn dough used as a base for *arepas*, *tortillas*, porridges, and so on. You make it at home but some natural food stores have started carrying it already made.

Mirin—A sweet wine made from rice and used in cooking.

Miso—A salty paste made from fermented soybeans with or without grains. Many varieties are available (see *Soups* chapter).

Mochi—Cakes made from pounded sweet rice which are dried and later used in a variety of dishes. It can be made at home or purchased in a natural food store. Make sure to get the brown rice variety instead of the white.

Mugicha—Tea made from roasted barley.

Natto—Stringy, fermented soybeans which when mixed with scallions, *tamari* soy sauce, grated ginger, and *daikon*, makes an excellent companion to a bowl of rice. The taste for it has to be acquired for some people. A good source of protein. It can be homemade or store bought.

Nishime—A method of cooking vegetables with a minimal amount of water.

Nori—A variety of sea vegetable which comes pressed into thin paper-like sheets. It can be used as a garnish, a cover for *sushi* and rice balls, and also as a condiment.

Norimaki—A type of *sushi* which is made by rolling *nori*, rice, and vegetables together into a long roll with a *sushi* mat.

Ohagi—Little balls of cooked, sweet rice which can be covered with seeds, nuts, or *azuki* beans, among other things.

Ojiya—A porridge of soft rice, vegetables, and *miso* (sea salt or *tamari* soy sauce can substituted for the *miso*).

Sea salt—Salt from the sea, much healthier than commercial land salt which contains iodine, sugar, and chemicals.

Seitan—Wheat gluten which has been boiled (and optionally deep-fried as well) with *tamari* soy sauce, *kombu*, and water. It is a good replacement for meat.

Shiitake—A variety of dried mushroom which is helpful in breaking down animal fats within the body. It is used as a soup stock or in vegetable dishes.

Shio kombu—A condiment made from *kombu* and *tamari* soy sauce.

Shiso—Beefsteak plant leaves which are pickled with *umeboshi* plums for added color. It strengthens blood quality, and can be used as a condiment.

Soba—Japanese buckwheat noodles.

Somen—An extremely thin variety of Japanese wheat noodles.

Suribachi—A ceramic bowl with grooves, used with a pestle for grinding and puréeing.

Sushi—Rice formed into little balls and topped with fish or vegetables, as well as rolls (*norimaki*) made from *nori*, rice, and vegetables.

Sushi mat—Bamboo mat used for making *norimaki sushi*.

Takuan—*Daikon* rice-bran pickles.

Tamari—A name given to naturally made soy sauce to differentiate it from the commercially made, chemicalized ones.

Tekka—A strong condiment made out of burdock, carrots, lotus root, ginger, *miso*, and sesame. Available in natural food stores.

Tempeh—Cakes of fermented soybeans, used widely in Indonesia, and available in natural food stores. A good source of protein.

Tofu—A white cake made from soybeans and water, also known as bean curd, available fresh or dried.

Udon—Japanese wheat noodles.

Umeboshi—Salty pickled plums. Helps cleanse the blood and aids digestion.

Wakame—A thin, leafy variety of sea vegetable.

Yannoh—Grain beverage sometimes used as a coffee substitute—made from five different grains.

Bibliography

Macrobiotic Health Education Series

Kushi, Michio. *A Natural Approach: Allergies*. Edited by Mark Mead and John D. Mann. Tokyo: Japan Publications, Inc., 1985.

———. *A Natural Approach: Diabetes and Hypoglycemia*. Edited by John D. Mann. Tokyo: Japan Publications, Inc., 1985.

———. *A Natural Approach: Infertility and Reproductive Disorders*. Edited by Charles Millman and Phillip Jannetta. Tokyo: Japan Publications, Inc., 1987.

———. *A Natural Approach: Obesity, Weight Loss and Eating Disorders*. Edited by John D. Mann. Tokyo: Japan Publications, Inc., 1987.

———. *A Natural Approach: Stress and Hypertension*. Edited by Mark Mead. Tokyo: Japan Publications, Inc., 1988.

Macrobiotic Food and Cooking Series

Kushi, Aveline. *Cooking for Health: Allergies*. Edited by Rosalind Rhodes. Tokyo: Japan Publications, Inc., 1985.

———. *Cooking for Health: Diabetes and Hypoglycemia*. Edited by Rosalind Rhodes. Tokyo: Japan Publications, Inc., 1985.

———. *Cooking for Health: Infertility and Roproductive Disorders*. Edited by Helaine Honig. Tokyo: Japan Publications, Inc., 1987.

———. *Cooking for Health: Obesity, Weight Loss and Eating Disorders*. Edited by Helaine Honig. Tokyo: Japan Publications, Inc., 1987.

———. *Cooking for Health: Stress and Hypertension*. Edited by Sarah Lapenta. Tokyo: Japan Publications, Inc., 1988.

Cookbooks

Aihara, Cornellia. *Macrobiotic Kitchen*. Tokyo: Japan Publications, Inc., 1983.

———. *The Do of Cooking*, Chico. Calif.: George Ohsawa Macrobiotic Foundation, 1972.

Esko, Edward and Wendy. *Macrobiotic Cooking for Everyone*. Tokyo: Japan Publications, Inc., 1980.

Esko, Wendy. *Introducing Macrobiotic Cooking*. Tokyo: Japan Publications, Inc., 1978.

Estella, Mary. *Natural Foods Cookbook: Vegetarian Dairy-free Cuisine*. Tokyo: Japan Publications, Inc., 1985.

Kushi, Aveline. *How to Cook with Miso*. Tokyo: Japan Publications, Inc., 1978.

Kushi, Aveline, with Alex Jack. *Aveline Kushi's Complete Guide to Macrobiotic Cooking for Health, Harmony, and Peace*. N. Y.: Warner Publishing Co., 1984.

Kushi, Aveline, with Wendy Esko. *The Changing Seasons Macrobiotic Cookbook*. Wayne, N. J.: Avery Publishing Group, 1984.

Ohsawa, Lima. *Macrobiotic Cuisine*. Tokyo: Japan Publications, Inc., 1984.

Other Macrobiotic or Related Books

Aihara, Herman. *Basic Macrobiotics*. Tokyo: Japan Publications, Inc., 1985.

Brown, Virginia, with Susan Stayman. *Macrobiotic Miracle: How a Vermont Family Overcame Cancer*. Tokyo: Japan Publications, Inc., 1985.

Dufty, William. *Sugar Blues*. New York: Warner, 1975.

Heidenry, Carolyn. *An Introduction to Macrobiotics: A Beginner's Guide to the Natural Way of Health*. Brookline Mass.: Aladdin Press, 1984.

———. *Making the Transition to a Macrobiotic Diet*. Brookline, Mass.: Aladdin Press, 1984.

Kohler, Jean and Mary Alice. *Healing Miracles from Macrobiotics*. West Nyack, N.Y.: Parker, 1979.

Kotzsch, Ronald E. *Macrobiotics: Yesterday and Today*. Tokyo: Japan Publications, Inc., 1985.

Kushi, Aveline. *Lessons of Day and Night*. Wayne, N. J.: Avery Publishing Group, 1984.

Kushi, Michio. *The Book of Dō-In: Exercise for Physical and Spiritual Development*. Tokyo: Japan Publications, Inc., 1979.

Kushi, Michio. *The Book of Macrobiotics* (Revised edition), Tokyo: Japan Publications, Inc., 1987.

———. *Cancer and Heart Disease: The Macrobiotic Approach to Degenerative Disorders* (Revised edition), Tokyo: Japan Publications, Inc., 1985.

———. *The Era of Humanity*. Edited by Sherman Goldman. Brookline, Mass.: East West Journal, 1980.

———. *How to See Your Health: The Book of Oriental Diagnosis*. Tokyo: Japan Publications, Inc., 1980.

———. *Macrobiotic Home Remedies*. Edited by Marc Van Cauwenberghe. Tokyo: Japan Publications, Inc., 1985.

———. *Natural Healing through Macrobiotics*. Tokyo: Japan Publications, Inc., 1987.

———. *Your Face Never Lies*. Wayne, N.J.: Avery Publishing Group, 1983.

Kushi, Michio and Aveline. *Macrobiotic Pregnancy and Care of the Newborn*. Tokyo: Japan Publications, Inc., 1984.

———. *Macrobiotic Child Care & Family Health*. Tokyo: Japan Publications, Inc., 1986.

Kushi, Michio, with Alex Jack. *The Cancer Prevention Diet*. N. Y.: St. Martin's Press, 1983.

———. *Diet for a Strong Heart: Michio Kushi's Macrobiotic Dietary Guidelines for the Prevention of High Blood Pressure, Heart Attack, and Stroke*. New York: St. Martin's Press, 1985.

Kushi, Michio and the East West Foundation. *Cancer and Heart Disease: The Macrobiotic Approach to Degenerative Disorders*. Edited by Edward Esko. Tokyo: Japan Publications, Inc., 1982.

Mendelsohn, Robert, S. *Confessions of a Medical Heretic*. Chicago: Contemporary Books, 1979.

———. *Male Practice*. Chicago: Contemporary Books, 1980.

Nussbaum, Elaine, *Recovery: From Cancer to Health Through Macrobiotics.* Tokyo: Japan Publications, Inc., 1985.

Ohsawa, George. *Cancer and the Philosophy of the Far East.* Oroville, Calif.: George Ohsawa Macrobiotic Foundation, 1971.

Ohsawa, George, with William, Dufty. *You Are All Sanpaku.* N. Y.: University Books, 1965.

Sattilaro, Anthony, with Tom Monte. *Recalled by Life: The Story of My Recovery from Cancer.* Boston: Houghton-Mifflin, 1982.

Tara, William. *Macrobiotics and Human Behavior.* Tokyo: Japan Publications, Inc., 1985.

Index